DIABETES AND YOUR TEENAGER

Bonnie Estridge and Jo Davies

Thorsons

An Imprint of HarperCollins*Publishers*

For Claire, who's been there,
Suzy, who's nearly there,
and Hannah,
who doesn't have diabetes,
but has taught us a lot
about teenagers.

Thorsons
An Imprint of HarperCollins*Publishers*
77–85 Fulham Palace Road
Hammersmith, London W6 8JB
1160 Battery Street
San Francisco, California 94111–1213

Published by Thorsons 1996
1 3 5 7 9 10 8 6 4 2

© Bonnie Estridge and Jo Davies 1996

Bonnie Estridge and Jo Davies assert the moral right
to be identified as the authors of this work

A catalogue record for this book
is available from the British Library

ISBN 0 7225 3180 X

Printed in Great Britain by
Caledonian International Book Manufacturing Ltd, Glasgow

DIABETES AND YOUR TEENAGER

CONTENTS

ACKNOWLEDGEMENTS

The authors would like to say a special thank you to Roma Starosolsky, Senior Dietitian at Charing Cross Hospital, for her invaluable help.

We would also like to thank the following people for their help, support and encouragement:

the BDA Medical and Scientific Section
Chris Butler
Kate Campbell
Gloria Ferris
Vanessa Hilton
Graham Hood and Vanessa Hebditch at the BDA
Wanda Whiteley
Amanda Cranston.

Very special thanks to the many teenagers and parents who responded to our survey, contributing experiences and advice that was invaluable to us and, we're sure, to those who read this book now and in the future.

FOREWORD

Any parent of a teenager knows that this is a time in their child's life when he or she is not wanting to be different from their peers. If their friends are following some new trend, they want to go along with it and while this will be a time of experimenting and pushing the boundaries it is not usually a time when doing something different from the rest of their friends – like injecting with insulin or eating regularly and sensibly – is appealing. For parents, understandably this can be a time of worry – their teenage child will want to join with friends in all sorts of activities, possibly experimenting with alcohol or drugs, staying out late (and even something as innocuous as a slumber party at a friend's house can present its problems), skipping a meal here and there or consuming a diet of burgers and cola.

This is a book which looks at all these issues and more and gives a practical plan of action. It is one that will really help parent and child work out their differences and provide a sensible plan of action to protect the health and wellbeing of the teenager with diabetes, while allowing him or her a good measure of independence. Bonnie Estridge – herself a mother of a teenager with diabetes – and Jo Davies will take the stress out of situations which would otherwise be fraught with worry and arguments. All those questions a parent or child will want to ask are answered simply and accurately – about insulin, puberty, diet, sport and a whole host of other issues and medical detail. With a wealth of information and a sensitive handling of the emotional issues involved, *Diabetes and Your Teenager* is a book I would recommend to any parent, teacher, youth worker or medic.

Graham Hood
Head of Youth and Family Services
British Diabetic Association

INTRODUCTION

The teenagers we are talking about in this book are no different to any other teenagers. They love rock music – the louder the better – they may wear an array of strange clothes and weird jewellery, their hair is sometimes styled in a way that makes them look like something from another planet. They can be selfish, vain, neurotic and insolent. They cannot understand why you worry when they stay out late or hang around with undesirable friends and they hate it when you nag them for not being able to get up in the morning. In short, the teenagers in this book have the same rites of passage as any other teenager. The only difference is that they have diabetes.

Your son or daughter may have had diabetes for some years or may have just developed it; adolescence is a peak time for the onset of this condition. At the time of writing, there are 20,000 people under the age of 20 registered in the UK with insulin-dependent diabetes, and 15,800 are over the age of 10. The number of new diagnoses is increasing and the figures for the last decade are double those of the previous one, with 3,000 new cases being diagnosed annually, although it is not known why this should be.

It's perhaps not surprising that puberty is the peak time for children of either sex to develop the condition, as a massive hormonal upheaval is going on in the body. The teenager's reaction to looking after themselves and coping with the regime of insulin and regular meals is variable and, of course, depends entirely on the individual (and, to a certain extent, your response towards them). Your teenager may cope extremely well and take the required discipline in his or her stride. On the other hand, it may be bitterly resented and the teenage years – a stressful enough time for any parent – may be a nightmare of worry and uncertainty.

However well your son or daughter copes with diabetes, it is only natural that they will try to push the barriers to varying degrees so that they are able to live as normal a life as possible; they do not want to be seen by their peers as 'different' in any way. This is totally understandable, yet you know that the way ahead is littered with potential problems. No parent of a teenage child with diabetes can simply bury their head in the sand and hope these problems will simply 'go away' – they won't. All-night parties, too much sleep, too little sleep, eating an exclusive diet of junk food, not eating at all, sex, smoking, alcohol and drugs . . . It's no use simply saying 'don't' because the chances are they will experiment, follow their peers and take chances.

The purpose of this book is to inform and educate parents about every facet of how diabetes affects being a teenager; what to expect when they do push the barriers, how to help them get through these difficult years – in short, forewarned is forearmed. We want to help you, as parents, by arming you with the knowledge you need to handle explosive issues. We hope you will then feel able to educate your child on how to cope with having diabetes while steering them along the bumpy road of being a teenager. By addressing all the relevant issues and incorporating the experiences of other parents and teenagers who have already been on this difficult journey, you should feel confident and able to handle situations if and when they should arise.

One real worry many parents express is that they are not doing everything that is possible for their child simply because they are in the dark about so many aspects of how their teenager's behaviour may affect their diabetes (and vice versa). We hope that this book will give you all the support and information you need to banish this worry from your mind.

Do you belong to the British Diabetic Association (BDA)? If

not, now is the time to join! The BDA is a huge organization that provides invaluable links for both you, as a parent, and your teenager. The network of support groups around the country will enable you to meet or contact other parents who have a child with diabetes and the teenagers themselves can benefit enormously from the various youth schemes, weekends and holidays that the BDA organizes. The information, help and advice it offers is inestimable – there is always someone who will listen.

Note that, for reasons of convenience, in writing this book we refer to the teenager as 'he' or 'she' in alternate chapters.

Chapter 1

ABOUT DIABETES

If your child has had diabetes for some time and is now approaching adolescence, you are no doubt reading this book with apprehension, wondering what on earth the teenage years will bring. Even when a child does not have diabetes, the teens can be a pretty torturous time – enough to test the mettle of the least faint-hearted of parents. If your teenager has been diagnosed as having diabetes recently, then your bewilderment may be total; just as you were struggling to understand the formally precious little poppet who appears to have undergone a complete personality transplant overnight, along comes this devastating blow. Your child has a serious and potentially life-threatening condition that can only be controlled by routine, sensible diet and discipline. How can he possibly cope? And – most importantly for you – how can you help without being seen to be more of a worrying nag or heavy authoritarian than he already thought you were?

We both have personal knowledge of just how harrowing the teens – with or without diabetes – can be. One of us clearly remembers the reverberations of her own diabetic younger sister's adolescent years. The other has a rebellious teenage daughter (who does not have diabetes) whose hair-raising escapades are followed with total admiration by her younger, pre-teen sister (who does).

However, in an extensive survey of teenagers with diabetes and their parents we were happily surprised at just how well the vast majority were coping. The parents tended to take an unobtrusive but supportive role, though they admitted that they worried and often cajoled if they felt their child was being a little too laid back about their condition. The teenagers themselves gave an overall impression of being a well-balanced, contented bunch who were rational and wise to the needs of their own bodies. They simply get on with life, treating diabetes as an inconvenience rather than a major hurdle. Many commented that they would not be the people they are today without diabetes. As 15-year-old Hayley stated, 'My diabetes revolves around me, not me around my diabetes. I feel great about my life . . . and that includes my diabetes'. So, we hope that the very positive advice from our parents and teenagers running through this book will help and encourage you and that you will also gain knowledge from any less fortunate experiences.

Background Information

It's important to understand exactly what diabetes is and why, if left untreated, it is such a dangerous condition. It's also important to appreciate that it is a condition which can quickly be brought under control by a tried and tested medical method for which there is no 'alternative' substitute.

Essentially, diabetes results from an inability of the pancreas to produce a hormone called insulin, which is essential for processing glucose (sugar) in the body. Normally, insulin is made in the pancreas (a gland lying close to the stomach and liver), but in someone with diabetes, the pancreas fails to produce any (or enough) insulin. So, instead of being stored and used by the body for energy, the glucose remains in the blood. Eventually, glucose spills over into the urine and this is often how diabetes is diagnosed. If left untreated, a person with diabetes will become weak and eventually die because their body is not receiving energy from glucose, which is essential to keep it going.

Your teenager may (but probably won't!) be interested to learn that there is a fair amount of historical significance attached to diabetes. It is certainly not an illness of modern times and has been identified as a serious malady for thousands of years.

In 1550 BC, *Papyrus Ebers*, the first recorded ancient Egyptian medical document, describes the illness as originating from the East and Middle East and prescribes 'ground dragon's blood, onions and flaxseed boiled with honey and oil' as a cure for the trademark symptom – excessive urination.

The full name of the condition – diabetes mellitus – comes from the Greek language and means 'fountain of honey'. Indeed, medical practitioners of the time would taste the sickly sweet urine that is passed when there is a high level of glucose in the blood by way of a diagnostic test! Thankfully, these days we have the technology to test urine and blood without this being necessary, but, before it was available, tasting it was a benchmark test and, indeed, went on for centuries. In 1679, Thomas Willis, physician to King Charles II, described the taste of diabetics' urine as 'wonderfully sweet', but the condition that caused it 'the pissing evil'.

Theories on diet abounded for years, though with no success, and it became clear that near-starvation was the only short-term alternative to alleviate symptoms. The unfortunate sufferers eventually died anyway from malnutrition so the theorists had no real answer to the problem. It was only relatively recently – in the late nineteenth century – that doctors discovered that when a dog's pancreas was removed this produced symptoms of diabetes. This provided the first important clue to the condition. However, no one knew at that time which ingredient in the pancreas was missing in people who had diabetes and they continued to die from lack of real knowledge, although intolerance of sweet or starchy foods (carbohydrates) seemed to play a vital role.

In 1914, experimental evidence suggested that by allowing the patient only whisky and coffee (providing some calories and comfort!) until no glucose could be detected in the urine, then reintroducing low quantities of carbohydrate in the form of boiled vegetables plus fat and protein, levels could be raised cautiously to a point where glucose in the urine did not reappear. This new treatment was deemed successful and so practised until the discovery of insulin by Frederick Banting and Charles Best in 1921.

Scientists Banting and Best discovered the importance of insulin while working through their summer holidays at the University of Toronto. It was known that the pancreas releases essential digestive juices that enable food to be absorbed into the body, but Banting and Best's critical finding was that the pancreas also produces various hormones that flow directly into the bloodstream. The most crucial of these hormones is insulin because of its aforementioned role in helping convert sugar from the food we eat into energy and storing it in cells around the body. Knowing what insulin does meant that the lack of it could then be seen to be the key to overcoming diabetes. An insulin replacement (at that time taken from the pancreas of pigs or cows) was first given to a 14-year-old boy who lay dying of diabetes in a hospital near to the University of Toronto. He made a remarkable recovery and insulin replacement was acclaimed to be a miracle discovery.

Banting and Best had found that when there is a lack of insulin, the body cannot make the correct use of sugar and so the level of glucose in the blood rises well above the normal limit (this is known as hyperglycaemia). Soon, the blood glucose rises so high that it spills over into the kidneys and is passed out in the urine, thus creating the 'fountain of honey'. Eventually, survival becomes impossible as there is not enough insulin to convert glucose into energy and the body begins to 'feed from itself' by breaking down fat and protein in a hopeless attempt to obtain energy. Unless insulin is replaced, therefore, serious illness is inevitable at such an advanced stage and an array of unpleasant symptoms present themselves.

There are certain tell-tale signs of diabetes, but it's quite possible for a busy teenager to ignore or explain away such symptoms to himself or his parents when it's not 'socially convenient' to be ill. The signs and the explanations are like the following.

- Unquenchable thirst. 'It's so hot at the moment.'
- Endless trips to the toilet. 'I'm drinking so much because it's hot.'
- Recurrent bouts of thrush (itching genitals). 'Must be that new shower gel I've been using.'

- A strange smell on the breath rather like peardrops or nail-polish remover. 'Must be something I ate.'
- Lack of energy. 'So much homework . . . '
- Blurred vision from glucose filling the lens of the eye and causing distortion. 'Maybe I need glasses.'

If these symptoms went unheeded and the condition progressed, then, sooner or later, it would become obvious that something serious was amiss. Severe tiredness, inexplicably fast weight-loss, weakness and extreme irritability would follow, caused by the 'fat and protein meltdown'. The peardrop-smelling breath is because of a substance called acetone and this occurs because of the presence of ketones, which are poisonous chemicals in the blood. At this stage, the build-up of ketones, coupled with drastic loss of weight and absence of energy, progresses rapidly to coma and, if left untreated, to death. However, it's quite incredible how quickly symptoms disappear and a seriously ill patient is restored to former health once he is treated with insulin.

One mother recalls:

> Heather looked pale and alarmingly thin over quite a short period of time and I began to wonder if she was becoming anorexic even though she did appear to be eating normally. She had never complained about being thirsty or anything else for that matter . . . probably because she was out so much I hardly saw her. Then one morning I went into her room and she was very drowsy, could hardly get out of bed. I called the doctor immediately and she was admitted to hospital virtually in a coma. Her recovery was rapid but I blamed myself for a long time – I should have been more vigilant.

Whether your child reaches the stage where he is admitted to hospital or is treated as an out-patient (this depends on how ill he becomes and/or the type of diabetes service you have in your area), both you as parents and he will be given intensive education as to how diabetes can be managed at home. This involves explaining how to inject insulin and do home blood tests. You will be told that the goal now is to keep blood glucose levels within a 'normal' range. In a person who does *not* have diabetes, the range is very narrow. Even after meals, it usually stays between 3.5 and 8 mmol/l, unless severe shock or undue stress causes it to rise. However, the sometimes wild blood glucose fluctuations seen in a person with diabetes would never be found in a person without it. Without insulin in the body, the amount of glucose in the blood can rise to ten or more times the normal level. Insulin replacement is intended to try and keep the blood glucose within a normal – or at least acceptable – range. Your child will be urged to aim for between 4 and 10 mmol/l by recording finger-prick test results, watching his diet, adjusting and injecting insulin according to his needs.

There will be a number of medical staff involved in the care of your son or daughter and all young people should be under the care of a hospital, whether treatment started at home as an out-patient or in hospital. The hospital will have a clinic specifically for the treatment of people with diabetes and your child will be asked to attend as an out-patient for check-ups at various intervals.

The doctor at the head of the 'team' may be a diabetologist or an endocrinologist (specializing in the system of glands in the body that give out hormones). Some older teenagers may be somewhat put out to find that they are under the care of a paediatrician (children's doctor), but some paediatricians continue to see young adults until they are 20.

In certain cases, the family GP may take charge. The doctor looking after your son or daughter will work out the initial treatment, at first altering insulin doses – sometimes frequently – to get the blood glucose down to normal levels.

The diabetes specialist nurse (who usually works only in the field of diabetes, but who may also be a health visitor) will also be closely involved in treatment and it will be she who helps your son or daughter learn about diabetes and advises on the practicalities of day-to-day living.

The relationship between your child and the diabetes specialist nurse is most important; she is your main link with the hospital, the one who helps sort out problems and provides a shoulder to cry on, if needed. In the early days following diagnosis, you may wish she was living with you permanently as there are so many questions you need to ask, but, as confidence grows – and it does – the teenager will become his own expert.

The other important member of the diabetes team is the dietitian, who will probably be based in the hospital (although some are community-based). The dietitian will assess if your son or daughter is eating the right foods and advise how their diet can be modified if this is necessary. Diet is, of course, one of the biggest problems that parents imagine will face the teenager (bearing in mind their love of fast foods), but you will find out that a 'diabetes diet' – if it can even be called that – is normal, healthy eating and simply follows the Government's recommendations for the population as a whole. A change of habits will be advised if many sugary or fatty foods are consumed, but this is good advice for everyone, whether or not they have diabetes. Later in this book we go on to explain every aspect of treatment and diet.

'Why Me?'

This is a question your son or daughter is bound to ask. The fact is, no one really knows why diabetes strikes some people and not others. Your son or daughter may be surprised (and perhaps rather comforted) to know that the condition is becoming increasingly common. Everyone seems to know someone who has diabetes and it should be made perfectly clear to your child that having diabetes is nothing to be ashamed of.

Try to take a low-key approach to how you see treatment fitting into your teenager's life (we will discuss many aspects of this later). Injections and blood tests must now be fitted in routinely with everyday living, which is bound to be seen as a major upheaval and total inconvenience. If your attitude appears to reinforce this opinion, then he will simply find it harder to cope. Try to calmly explain that diabetes will not go away, but it need not take over his life and, indeed, will only do so if he allows it to. The key to smooth diabetes management is normality, and your teenager must now try to fit the treatment into his life and make it a normal part of day-to-day living. 'Try not to smother with kindness or treat them any differently . . . ', advises Maria, whose 16-year-old daughter has diabetes.

Try to explain to your child that he's not alone in his 'plight'. There are over 600,000 people in the UK alone registered as having diabetes (although not all of these are dependent on insulin). Type 1, or insulin-dependent diabetes, usually occurs between between birth and the age of 40. Those with Type 1 diabetes eventually produce little or no insulin and will have to rely on treatment for the rest of their lives unless a complete cure is found. Right now, despite tremendous research activity into finding such a cure, one is not likely to be found in the near future. Older people who have Type 2, or non-insulin-dependent diabetes, still produce some insulin and are able to control their blood glucose by being careful with their diet, taking tablets or a combination of the two. There are an estimated 30 million people with diabetes worldwide and around 25 per cent of these are insulin-dependent. Fifteen-year-old David notes, 'It's hard, it's frustrating, it's horrible – but you have to live with it. There are hundreds of people just like you. They're coping, so get on with it!'

The incidence of insulin-dependent diabetes in children under 15 in the UK has doubled and 3,000 cases are now being diagnosed annually. But why? The fact that no one knows is worrying to say the least. It's true that certain families have a strong tendency to develop the condition, yet, in most new cases, parents cannot trace even one relative with diabetes on either side of the family. It must be likely, therefore, that many people carry a gene or susceptibility to diabetes and that there is a trigger factor that turns it into the full-blown illness. Indeed, young people often develop diabetes after a viral illness or infection and it is quite possible that a particular virus (as yet unidentified) is the cause. However, there is no such thing as a diabetes virus and it is impossible to 'catch' it from someone else. Diabetes will only occur in a person who already has the tendency and then catches the 'trigger' virus. The chances of your child passing on diabetes to future children are 1 in 20 for a man and 1 in 50 for a woman, yet, even in cases where both parents have diabetes, many children never develop the disease.

Sometimes it is suggested that diabetes has developed as a result of a shock to the system (such as an accident) or some kind of major upheaval. Although a shock in itself cannot actually cause diabetes, it may be true that emotional stress or trauma could provoke an increase in blood glucose, which, in turn, could trigger the diabetes that was already developing. It is possible that the cause of diabetes may be environmental, but a hard and fast yes or no answer to this idea, unfortunately, seems to be a long way off.

There are certain 'peak' times for people to develop diabetes. Hospitals and clinics find that the number of cases rises significantly during the late winter months. As more colds and infections are around in late winter, this would seem to back up the virus/trigger theory. Also, as we mentioned in the Introduction, puberty is a peak time for children of either sex to develop diabetes and this is almost certainly due to the enormous metabollic upheaval that occurs in adolescence.

At some point, your teenager may lay the blame on you for their diabetes. An accusation such as this is naturally most disturbing, but it is important to try not to allow this to upset you too much. You are bound to worry that something you may have done in the past – such as allowing your child too many sweets or junk foods from an early age – may be to blame, yet doctors and scientists do not know if diet is a cause of insulin-dependent diabetes. So, you can rest assured that there is nothing you or anyone else could have done to prevent your child from having diabetes and nothing you may have done would have caused it. Take a deep breath and let the recriminations wash over you as it's natural that your child needs someone to vent his anger on and you need to be able to listen sympathetically, but try to make him understand that nobody is to blame. Remember, too, that teenagers invariably put the onus on parents for their problems and if it wasn't diabetes it would be something like 'It's your fault I'm so fat/spotty/short . . . '. Unfortunately, as a parent of a teenager, it's often your role in life – for a few years anyway – to be a verbal punchbag!

Despite how commonplace diabetes is becoming, there is still a certain amount of ignorance about it (it's amazing how many people think that eating sugar will cause someone with diabetes to fall into a coma immediately!) So, the more people can be educated as to what diabetes really is, the better. 'I don't want people to think I'm a freak!', is a typical teenage protest, and sometimes a reason for hiding their diabetes from friends. You must make it quite clear that nobody will find anything odd about them so long as they explain that they have diabetes and what it's all about. But they are far more likely to be thought of as a 'freak' (or just plain stupid) if friends are left in the dark as to what is going on and find themselves in a situation they cannot handle (a bad hypo for instance). Otherwise, how could they possibly know that the incoherantly mumbling person who appeared perfectly normal one moment is not now roaring drunk but needs to eat something sugary.

A teenager who has had diabetes for some time will have to confront the demands of finally taking responsibility for himself if he wants to break away from his parents' apron-strings. Until this time, the main worries of diet, insulin and so on will have rested with the parents and the full implications of the condition have to be realized and dealt with from then on by the teenager. He may have come to rely on you a bit too much. One mother was very worried that her 13-year-old son still insisted she do his injections and therefore had little in the way of a social life. However, not long after she had reported her concern to the doctor, Paul found a girlfriend and, not wanting mum to accompany him on dates, suddenly took over everything for himself. And, no, he didn't ask his girlfriend to do the injections!

It's not easy to adjust to the extra responsibility put on a teenager's shoulders by their diabetes and, as self-discipline is pretty foreign to any teenager, it's hardly surprising that some totally reject the regime. But, you have to remember that rebellion usually goes hand in hand with being a teenager and it would be strange – even a little worrying perhaps – if there were no such period of rebellion, which, in this case, would almost certainly be against the diabetes and all it entails. Later in this book we shall be covering the invaluable help that a teenager with diabetes can gain from talking over their problems with a psychologist who specializes in counselling children with diabetes. They might not like the idea at first, but, once cajoled into going, it's amazing how they begin to feel a burden lifting. The same applies to the special youth schemes and holidays run by the BDA, where teenagers can meet others of their own age with diabetes. An overwhelming number of youngsters in our survey said they had benefited immensely from these opportunities, and we cover this subject in greater detail later on.

When children with diabetes reach adulthood, there is no reason for them not to marry and have healthy children of their own. The careful handling of the situation should resolve problems in the teens and your child will then find that there is little which is insurmountable. It is absolutely possible for him to lead a normal and fulfilled life, as many top athletes, actors, professionals and others who have diabetes will confirm.

'It's not the end of the world,' says 16-year-old Sarah. 'And there's no use trying to fight or rebel against something that will be with you for the rest of your life or until a cure is discovered. If anyone tells you you're not normal, challenge them to define "normal" for you.'

Sarah's positive beliefs are echoed by Anna, aged 12: 'Injecting can be a pain. But, overall, diabetes has made my life more interesting. If you're somewhere and there's an awkward silence, it's something to talk about. It's certainly helped me to grow up.'

Chapter 2

THE UPHEAVAL OF PUBERTY

The Changing Body

Although children are not 'officially' teenagers until they hit that magic thirteenth birthday, puberty is usually well under way by this time. The average child will have started the internal biological development that heralds adolescence by around nine or ten, stimulated by a dramatic increase in sex hormones. Although certain outward signs may not be apparant for several years, a classic feature of early puberty is a major growth spurt resulting from the sudden increase in growth hormone. During this time of rapid change, the average adolescent grows around 30 cm (12 in) and may put on up to 13 kg (2 stone) in weight. In girls, this growth spurt occurs right at the beginning of puberty whereas in boys it does not occur until about two years later – hence the problem of 12- and 13-year-old girls complaining that they find boys of their own age 'much too short'. Indeed, some girls find themselves towering over their peers (of either sex) at 11 or 12 only to find themselves the shortest of the group at 14 or 15.

The age at which individuals begin to display outward signs of development depends, to some extent, on genetic influences (a girl often starts her periods at the same age her mother did, for example). However, your son or daughter will find that there are no hard and fast rules as to when the body starts changing into that of an adult and the differences between and even within the sexes are great. Some girls begin to show signs of puberty as early as 8, others as late as 13 – some even later. Some boys are tall and their voices have broken at 12 whereas some may not look anything close to 'manly' at 16. If your child was diagnosed as having diabetes just before puberty or her diabetes was poorly controlled and blood glucose levels were high, the onset of puberty may have been delayed for these reasons.

As growth and sex hormones counteract the effects of insulin, they will almost certainly cause glucose levels to be raised at certain times. Growth hormone is secreted around the body in surges rather than as a steady trickle. A graph of growth hormone levels in the blood over 24 hours shows wildly uneven peaks and troughs, which are so unpredictable that it's hardly surprising that equally uneven peaks and troughs of glucose levels follow in their wake. Your priority now is to encourage your child to try and gain as much control over her diabetes as is possible. Some young people are able to control their blood glucose far more successfully than others. To an extent, this depends on their metabolism and on how disciplined they are about balancing insulin with meals and exercise. Of course, their attitude towards their diabetes is really the key to successful blood glucose management. Discipline is not a virtue usually associated with teenagers, but a good understanding of the mechanics of diabetes control, coupled with the hi-tech aids available today, will go a long way towards helping them *want* to take care of themselves so that they are able to lead a completely normal life. See Chapter 3 for detailed information on controlling blood glucose levels.

From Girl to Woman

Although internal changes may have been taking place for some time, the first outward sign of a girl turning into a woman is a marked swelling around the breast. This is not to be confused with enlargement of the breast itself, for this is just fatty tissue and rather more connected with weight gain. Pink, sometimes tender 'buds' are the real indication that the breast is developing, although full development takes some years and it is only when the breast becomes full and solid that the transition is complete.

The appearance of sparse pubic hair is the next stage, and during this time the growth spurt will have begun. An increase in fat is often noticeable around the hips, buttocks, arms and thighs, with muscle developing to replace this 'puppy fat' at a later stage (although girls tend to lose less fat than boys, which is a normal part of their shape filling out). The teens are a crucial time for try-ing to keep weight under control and girls in particular tend to worry that the shape confronting them in the mirror is not con-forming to society's 'ideal'.

If your daughter is overweight and wants to diet, there is no reason why she should not do this, so long as she talks to her diet-itian. This way, a safe method that brings results can be fitted around her insulin injections. If there are any signs that your son or daughter has realized that constantly high sugars lessen the appetite for food (leading to weight loss) and so is tempted to drop the dose of insulin (or even go without it completely), then you must try to put a stop to this immediately; it is dangerous. Suggest a visit to the clinic to discuss a sensible way of dieting and insulin reduction with the dietitian and diabetes specialist nurse.

Obviously, if your child is seriously overweight then a diet is of real importance, not only for the sake of vanity and self-esteem but also for future health. However, teenagers (and it's usually girls) who are *not* overweight and appear to be overly obsessed with the shape of their bodies should be watched extremely carefully for signs of eating disorders. In Chapter 6, we cover the whole busi-ness of weight problems, eating disorders and diet solutions in depth.

Although a girl's internal sexual organs have been growing for some time – in an average child this starts by nine or ten – the out-ward signs of development may not show for several years. The start of periods, or menstruation (the menarche), does not usually occur for two to three years after initial outward signs of puberty occur. A girl usually longs for her first period – a sign that she really is a woman, capable of bearing children. Once the novelty wears off, girls tend to take periods in their stride, merely seeing them as a minor inconvenience. Mothers need to be aware that their own attitude to periods may shape their daughters'. If you have always treated menstruation as some kind of dreadful monthly disaster, then your daughter is probably also going to see it as 'the curse'. If your attitude has been matter-of-fact and low-key, then she will react in the same way and treat periods as a natural part of being a woman.

In some girls with diabetes, blood glucose levels go crazy around 'that time of the month'. In some girls this leads to high glucose levels and in other girls low levels. It is not known exactly why there are two such diverse reactions to the same problem, but the same thing seems to happen every month to the same individual. Girls with (and without) diabetes often find that their appetite increases just before a period begins, which often leads to overeating and, in turn, to higher glucose levels. Tracey – now 21 – told us:

I'm quite used to it now, but when my periods started at 13 I could never understand why I wanted to binge like a maniac three or four days before my period. My blood sugars were sky-high and I found it very hard to control them at that time. By the time I was 17 or so, I didn't feel that terrible urge to eat . . . it went away and now I don't feel any different before a period and I don't need to adjust my insulin. I don't know why it suddenly stopped being like that . . .

Yet, some find that despite eating more, their levels are low. Teenage girls can suffer from premenstrual syndrome (PMS), but, unless the symptoms are particularly marked and only manifest themselves before a period, an uptight and bolshy daughter may just be par for the course rather than anything to do with her menstrual cycle. However, it's interesting that Dr Katharina Dalton (the UK's foremost authority on premenstrual syndrome) explains that the female hormone, progesterone, plays a part in regulating blood glucose levels. When progesterone levels drop in the days leading up to a period, many women who don't have diabetes and do not eat some starchy food every three hours find themselves experiencing symptoms similar to low glucose levels in diabetes. In her book *Once A Month* (Fontana, London, 1991), Dr Dalton advises women suffering from the classic PMS symptoms of irritability, headaches, drowsiness and general lack of energy to eat small portions of starchy foods at regular intervals. Perhaps it follows that if your daughter is displaying particularly antisocial behaviour patterns just before a period, it is a sign that her glucose levels are low and her insulin dose should be adjusted or starchy carbohydrate intake increased.

The only way to establish a pattern and deal with it is by regular blood testing in the days leading up to a period. If your daughter shows a regular pattern of high or low glucose levels connected with her periods, then she will need to raise or lower her insulin to balance her food accordingly, and then change the dose again once the period has arrived. It's worth remembering that girls' periods are often irregular for the first year or so after menstruation begins and this may cause difficulties in establishing a pattern of glucose levels. However, they will become more predictable with maturity. A 'regular' cycle is not necessarily one that has 28 days between the first day of each period; most cycles are anywhere in between 20 and 36 days, with 28 days merely being an 'average' statistic. Once your daughter's periods have settled down to the cycle that is regular for *her*, any problems of rising or falling glucose levels will become easier to deal with.

Incidentally, there is no 'right' age for menstruation to begin, but if there has been no sign of one by the time your daughter is 16, you should consult the doctor. The same applies if she has persistent missed periods (amenhorrea) and you are certain that she is not pregnant as poorly controlled diabetes can be a reason for this.

Periods are often accompanied by abdominal cramps. Exactly what causes these is not known for certain, although the main theory is that overproduction of prostaglandins (a hormone-like substance) causes the womb to contract and block the flow of blood. Most women have period cramps at some time, but these can vary from a dull ache to quite strong pain. However, if periods cause your daughter extreme discomfort (headaches, severe cramps, nausea and vomiting or bad backache), you should not assume this is 'normal'. It is called dysmenorrhoea and is often caused by hormone imbalance or an infection in the pelvic area. Problems causing severe period discomfort can all be treated, often by taking the Pill. However, your diabetes consultant will indicate whether or not this treatment would be suitable. Incidentally, blood glucose levels can be affected (that is, raised) by pain, as it is a form of stress.

From Boy to Man

Although boys begin their growth spurt considerably later than girls, once it does start, it is faster and carries on for longer. Whereas at 12 the average boy is smaller than his girl contemporaries, by 15 he is heavier, taller and stronger.

The first outward sign of male puberty is when the testicles become larger and noticeably drop between the legs. The sac that holds the testicles – the scrotum – becomes darker and some boys may notice swellings beneath their nipples (this nearly always disappears within a year). Greater hormonal activity in the testes produces the development of pubic hair and a light 'bumfluff' on the upper lip. The penis begins to grow and the voice begins to deepen with the accompanying embarrassing 'breaks' from high to low pitch.

The later signs of puberty in boys are bodily and facial hair becoming coarse and the stabilizing of the deep voice. With the hormone testosterone flowing in large amounts through the body, boys often have involuntary erections and, although they will have experienced erections since birth, they will now produce sperm and ejaculate. To many boys, this is often the most important sign of sexual maturity – in the same way periods are to girls.

Although your son will not have the problem of blood glucose levels reacting to monthly cycles, sex and growth hormones will still affect his metabolism and may raise his levels considerably. Increasing insulin to cope with this is vital. Exercise helps immensely and the more sport he wants to do, the better! This, of course, goes for girls as well, although teenage girls are notorious for suddenly dropping sports that they once adored, usually because they interfere with their social lives. Try to encourage your son or daughter to spend time doing physical exercise because, not only is it good for the blood glucose, it keeps them fit and stops them turning into couch potatoes! More about exercise in Chapter 5.

Emotional Issues

It's easy to blame all those circulating hormones for the classic rebellious, non-communicative behaviour of the average teenager, but, to a large extent, *is* the reason. Indeed, it would be rare for anyone to sail through such a dramatic physical change in their life without a wimper. Most adolescents are moody and have fluctuating emotions. They want to be seen as individuals and often push the goalposts of the limitations they see before them to see just how far they can go. As we discussed earlier, it's a rare teenager who does not go through some kind of rebellion, whether it's what time they should be home, how outrageous a hairstyle they can get away with, how loud they can play their music or how many unsuitable friends they can hang around with.

Diabetes is another factor in this equation and they may well alight on their diabetes as a weapon to use against you in the teenager v parent battle. A child who coped with her diabetes easily until the teens suddenly realizes that if she wants to be her own person and lead a completely normal life, she can no longer leave her parents to worry about her diet, insulin and so on. She must now take full responsibility for it all herself and the serious implications of the condition may hit her hard. She doesn't really want to 'go it alone' but knows she must, it scares her and perhaps she tries to reject her diabetes and any help you may offer, as one mother reports:

Claire had always accepted that she had diabetes and often told us she felt that it made her what she was . . . an individual. When she reached 13, all this changed. She didn't want to be that particular individual any longer . . . Life became very difficult for a couple of years until she accepted the help of the hospital psychologist, whose help we found inestimable.

If a child has had diabetes for some time, then friends are bound to know something about it. If she develops it during adolescence, she may decide to keep it a secret. One TV soap showed a teenage girl being caught injecting insulin by a friend, who assumed she was taking drugs. The girl with diabetes decided to keep up the facade of taking drugs as she assumed her friends would accept being a junkie as more cool than having diabetes. The TV soap handled the problem well as when her friends found out the truth, they felt betrayed by her lies. Lying about something so important, they pronounced, was distinctly *uncool.*

The shock of diagnosis during adolescence can affect the whole family, as Mark's mother, Barbara, found out.

Mark was 15 when he developed diabetes. He treated it with anger, frustration and disbelief. It was hard to tell whether his mood swings were from normal teenage behaviour or whether he was being affected by poor blood glucose levels . . . But he was very hard to live with at times!

Barbara tells us that, five years on, Mark has accepted his diabetes and has become far easier to live with.

He has realized that if he is going to enjoy his life in spite of having diabetes he must stop moaning and complaining 'why me?'. He has come to terms with the fact that it really isn't anyone's fault and he is getting on with his studies and trying to lead as full a social life as possible. He now knows he won't find life as free and easy as some of his friends, but he knows he is better off than many other people.

Obviously the teenage years are when the majority of school and social problems arise and we cover these in detail in Chapter 7.

Chapter 3

CONTROLLING
DIABETES

There is only one treatment for insulin-dependent diabetes and that is the replacement of insulin by injection; there is no alternative right now. Scientists constantly look for other ways of taking insulin, but a successful method remains elusive. Unfortunately, insulin cannot be taken in tablet form as it is a protein and would therefore be digested before reaching the bloodstream. You may have heard of older people with diabetes taking tablets, but these are not actually insulin. They are, in fact, drugs to stimulate the pancreas to produce more insulin. In older people who develop non-insulin-dependent diabetes, the pancreas is still able to produce *some* insulin. So, the action of the injected insulin in those who cannot produce insulin at all is to mimic the pancreas of a non-diabetic as closely as possible. For example, when someone who does *not* have diabetes eats, their blood glucose level rises, but the beta cells in the pancreas produce enough insulin to bring the glucose level back to normal. In a person *with* diabetes, however, this effect must be achieved by injecting insulin.

Some years ago, the treatment for diabetes was simply to take insulin to stay alive and hope for the best. There was no real way of telling precisely what effect the insulin was having on blood glucose levels except by testing the urine via a rather long-winded kind of chemical experiment. When doctors realized how important it was to monitor the level of glucose in the blood and control it, modern technology made it possible for this to be done simply and relatively cheaply at home without having to wait months between visits to the clinic when the random tests that were done at that time told the patient very little. Even 15 years ago, there was just not the technology we have now to give people with diabetes a real insight into their blood glucose levels.

There are various reasons for the importance of blood testing. First, it enables someone with diabetes to take immediate action by adjusting insulin doses accordingly to avoid hypos and hypers. Also, in the long term, doing this may well prevent damage to the body, known as 'diabetic complications' (which will be explained in detail in Chapter 4). Before we discuss these, however, you need to understand everything about insulin therapy and why it is so vital for your teenager to inject it regularly.

Taking Control

As we mentioned in the previous chapter, a normal blood glucose range in the non-diabetic is between 3.5 and 8 mmol/l. The measurement of millimoles per litre (mmol/l) is used throughout the EU and 4 mmol/l is the equivalent to a ¼ of a teaspoon of sugar dissolved in 1 litre (1¾ pints) of water. For your son or daughter to constantly aim for these levels would put him or her at risk of having frequent hypos and this certainly would compromise any bid for a normal lifestyle. Rather, consider blood glucose levels of between 4 and 10 mmol/l (the lower level before meals, the higher after) safe both from the point of view of lifestyle and lessening the risk of future complications. However, there is one time in a woman's life that blood glucose should be extremely tightly controlled, and that is before and during pregnancy – something we will discuss later in this book.

To achieve the required blood glucose levels, the dose and type of insulin needs to be balanced with food and exercise. This can be tricky for the teenager when you take everything into account – social life, sleeping habits and, of course, hormonal activity. But the difficulty of obtaining good control should not put you off trying or at least making sure the child fully understands why it's important to try himself. Insulin is measured in units and there are various types. Once injected, their action is intended to mimic the pancreas as far as possible. The different categories of insulin are described below, and your diabetes consultant will choose the best regime to fit in with your son or daughter's lifestyle.

Clear Insulin

Also called soluble, regular, short- or quick-acting, it is completely transparent in appearance and begins to work shortly after it has been injected. It peaks (which means it is most effective) between two and four hours after injecting. As blood glucose levels rise after eating food, this insulin works after a meal, such as breakfast. If your teenager is on multiple injections (three or four a day), then clear insulin only will be injected before meals and cloudy insulin only before bed.

Cloudy Insulin

Often called medium-acting or intermediate, this is opaque and looks much thicker than clear insulin. Once injected, it begins to work one to two hours later, peaking between six and eight hours after the injection. Cloudy insulin usually lasts 12 to 14 hours, but can work for up to 24 hours. Therefore, if it is injected before breakfast, it will start to work about mid morning and peak to coincide with the rise in blood glucose after lunch. It continues to work during the afternoon up until the evening meal and then begins to tail off. Another injection is then given before the evening meal. There are also some cloudy insulins known as slow- or long-acting that can last up to 36 hours. Medium- and long-acting insulins are often used in combination with clear insulin to cover blood glucose peaks and troughs throughout the day. This is known as free-mixing and can only be done if a syringe is used.

Fixed mixtures

Also called Bi-Phasic insulin, this is cloudy in appearance and is a mixture of short- and medium-acting insulin in one bottle. It comes in different ratios of clear to cloudy, such as 10/90, 20/80, 30/70, 40/60 and 50/50. For example, if you see a bottle with 30/70, it means the contents are 30 per cent clear and 70 per cent cloudy insulin, as the amount of short-acting, clear insulin is always written first.

The advantage of fixed mixtures is that they are ready-mixed and there is no need to use separate bottles of clear and cloudy. Many people use fixed mixtures in an insulin 'pen', which is ultra-convenient. The one disadvantage is that if extra short-acting insulin is required for one injection (perhaps to cover a large meal or during periods of illness), then it is not possible to increase just the short-acting component – the medium-acting component will be increased as well. To get around this, it would be necessary to have a separate injection of short-acting insulin at the same time or to use a syringe as opposed to a pen and add some extra units of short-acting insulin to the usual mixture. Incidentally, clear insulin should always be drawn up first.

Storing Insulin

The most suitable place to store insulin is in the fridge, away from the freezer compartment (it should be kept cool but never allowed to freeze). However, it is safe to keep insulin out of the fridge for a month, providing it is in a cool place and not exposed to direct heat, so windowsills, glove compartments of cars and so on must be avoided! It's actually better to keep the bottle or pen cartridge out of the fridge when in use as injecting insulin that has come straight from the fridge can be painful.

The type of insulin prescribed is designed to suit the needs of your teenager. If he developed diabetes as a child and has been used to two daily injections, you may find that his doctor advises increasing the number of injections to three or four a day. This does not mean your teenager's diabetes has become worse – there is no such thing as having diabetes 'worse' or 'better' than some-one else – it's all a matter of 'good' and 'bad' control. The aim in this case is to make your child's life more flexible now that he is in his teens and needs to become more independent. What consti-tutes the right amount of insulin, the mixture and the number of injections will vary from one person to another, and the doctor's aim is to control your son or daughter's diabetes in the most acceptable way possible.

The following are checklists for how to draw up insulin correctly.

Drawing Insulin Up Into a Syringe

How to draw up insulin from one bottle only.

- Check if you are using a 100-, 50- or 30-unit syringe. Each line on a 100-unit syringe equals 2 units of insulin, and each line on a 50- or 30-unit syringe is 1 unit.
- Check the expiry date on the bottle.
- Mix the insulin by rocking the bottle in your hands or tilting it up and down. Do this gently to prevent air bubbles forming, which could be difficult to get rid of.
- Take the syringe and pull back the plunger to draw air into it. Draw up the same amount of air as the dose of insulin to be taken.
- With the bottle upright (so the needle does not touch the insulin, which would create more bubbles) insert the needle through the rubber cap of the bottle and push the air in. It is not imperative to insert air into the bottle.
- Do not remove the needle, but turn the bottle upside down and make sure the tip of the needle is covered by the insulin.
- Hold onto the bottle and the syringe. Try to hold the bottle steady – if it moves around too much this may bend the needle. Pull out the plunger and the insulin will be drawn into the syringe. Draw up a little more insulin than you need.
- Remove the syringe from the bottle and, with the needle pointing upwards, gently tap the syringe and allow any air bubbles to rise to the top. Air bubbles are not dangerous as

such, but they will prevent the right amount being drawn up.
- Gently push the plunger to expel any air bubbles or any extra insulin. Make sure the top of the plunger in the syringe is in line with the amount of insulin required.

Mixing clear and cloudy insulin in the same syringe.

- Check the expiry dates on the bottles.
- Mix the cloudy insulin by rocking the bottle in your hands or gently tilting it up and down.
- Pull out the plunger of the syringe and draw up the same amount of air as the amount of *cloudy* insulin to be taken.
- Hold the bottle of cloudy insulin upright. Push the syringe into the bottle and inject the air in. Remove the syringe. You do not draw up any cloudy insulin at this stage.
- Now draw up the same amount of air as the amount of *clear* insulin required.
- Inject this air into the upright bottle of clear insulin. Turn the bottle upside down, make sure the tip of the needle is covered by the insulin, and the bottle is held steady. Draw up the clear insulin, a little more than you need. You always draw clear insulin into the syringe first.
- Remove the syringe from the bottle. With the needle upright, tap the syringe so the air bubbles rise to the top. Gently expel any air bubbles and any extra insulin. Make sure the top of the plunger in the syringe is in line with the amount of clear insulin required.
- Take the bottle of cloudy insulin (make sure it is properly mixed), insert the syringe, turn the bottle upside down, making sure the tip of the needle is covered by the insulin. Draw up the amount of cloudy insulin required. Do not forget you already have clear insulin in the syringe so you will have to add the amount of cloudy insulin on to that, so, if 4 units of clear and 10 of cloudy are needed, the plunger should be on the 14 unit line. If you draw up too much cloudy insulin by mistake, *do not* inject it back into the bottle, as you will be injecting back clear insulin too. Instead, *discard all the insulin and start again.*

Your doctor or diabetes nurse may suggest adding clear insulin to pre-mixed insulin if extra short-acting insulin is needed to cover a large meal. The procedure for this is the same as above, with the clear insulin always being drawn up into the syringe first.

Absorption Rates

Insulin is absorbed at different rates depending where it is injected. It is absorbed most quickly from the abdomen, then the arms, then the thighs and buttocks. Vigorous exercise also speeds up the rate of absorption, as does heat. So, it is wise for your teenager not to inject before a bath or shower as the warmth will make the blood vessels dilate and the insulin will be absorbed quicker, causing the blood glucose level to fall and this could lead to a hypo. Also, take care in hot weather as you might need to inject nearer mealtimes than during cooler times of the year.

Getting the Technique Right

The needles on the syringe and the pen are very short and the design ensures that there is no danger of hitting a major blood vessel. At the time of writing, even shorter and finer needles for pens have become available. The angle of the needle when going into the skin should be at 90 degrees to it, unless your teenager is very thin, in which case he should inject at a slant, at 45 degrees into the skin. Sometimes a little insulin leaks out, but the amount is minimal and so no more should be injected. The hole can be sealed by quickly pulling the skin to one side. A spot of blood (from a small capillary) is harmless, but may cause some bruising.

It is very important to keep changing sites, for repeatedly injecting into one place can cause the skin to become hard and lumpy and injecting into lumps can slow down the absorption rate of the insulin, resulting in bad control as more insulin is needed for anything at all to be absorbed. When looking for lumps, don't expect to see ones that are golf ball- or mosquito bite-size – they could almost be mistaken for a muscle as they are rather like smooth mounds in the beginning. But worse can follow, as Sarah remembers:

I was on 4 injections a day, taking 40 units at each injection. I had always injected in my legs, even as a child, and my thighs were so unsightly I was embarrassed to wear a swimsuit. The reason I kept injecting in my legs was because eventually the lumps caused the injections to become completely painless. I joined a new clinic and as my diabetic control was so erratic, the diabetes nurse suggested I change injection sites and suggested I reduce the amount of insulin at each injection. Because I had needed to give myself so much insulin through the lumps, I had some hypos when injecting the new site simply because I had no idea how much I really needed. I now take 18 units 4 times a day and my control is much better. I have left my legs alone and the lumps have almost gone.

Timing the Injections

Insulin should be injected 20 to 30 minutes before breakfast and the evening meal if taken as a mixture of clear and cloudy twice a day. This way, the insulin will start working as the food is being absorbed. If the time between the injection and the consumption of food is too long, then the insulin will have nothing to work on and the blood glucose level will fall low, resulting in a hypo either during or after the meal. Alternatively, if taken just before a meal, the insulin will start working *after* the food has been absorbed, causing a rise in blood glucose.

Given the erratic eating habits of the average teenager, you will know that it's not always possible for them to inject precisely 20 to 30 minutes before food, especially somewhere like a hamburger restaurant! In this case, it is a safer bet to inject as soon as the food arrives. If the injection has been done and a long wait does occur, some bread or a drink of fresh orange juice will usually save the situation until the meal arrives. If the injection is forgotten until the meal is over, there's no need to panic – it should be taken the minute it is remembered.

Once injected, the insulin peaks and falls coinciding with meal and snack times and the idea is that a balance between insulin and food should result, providing normal blood glucose levels.

But, can it really be that simple? Of course not – perfect results depend on several factors, some of which are predictable and some not. Let's look at how a mixture of clear and cloudy insulin works ifit is injected twice a day, either as a fixed mixture or 'free-mixed' (from separate clear and cloudy bottles).

Philip is on twice-daily injections. He takes his first injection before breakfast and the clear insulin starts to work as breakfast is being absorbed. It will peak to coincide with the rise in blood glucose levels after breakfast and throughout the morning. About mid morning, the cloudy insulin is beginning to work. Philip will need a snack at this time to prevent him having a hypo because of the amount of insulin in his bloodstream.

At lunchtime, the cloudy insulin is beginning to peak to co-incide with the rise in blood glucose after eating his meal. The cloudy insulin continues to work throughout the afternoon, so Philip will need another snack mid afternoon to stop him having a hypo again.

He takes his second injection before his evening meal and ensures he has a bedtime snack to prevent him having a hypo during the night.

There is a certain rigidity about injecting twice a day as a delayed meal or forgotten snack can result in a hypo, so timing is pretty important. Some teenagers will be happy with this, but there are those who will find it restricting as far as their social life is concerned and this may be a cause of frustration because they find their diabetes hard to control. As Ben says:

It can be a constant hassle. I don't want to keep eating snacks – I want to eat when I want to eat.

So Ben's best bet is to go on to four injections a day, which will solve the problem, and if he is not already using a pen injection device, then the doctor will no doubt suggest this to him.

Four-times-a-day Injections – How This Regime Works

Short-acting insulin is injected before breakfast, lunch and the evening meal and then medium- or long-acting before bed. In someone who does not have diabetes, the pancreas produces some background insulin all the time (the medium-acting insulin) and, each time they eat, there is a spurt of insulin (the short-acting kind). By mimicking this regime, the teenager can decrease or increase the amount of insulin depending on the size of the meal he is about to eat. If sport is on the agenda, he can take less insulin as he will be burning up more energy while exercising (see Chapter 5 for more on this).

It's very important to keep a close eye on blood glucose levels when treatment is changed. First, good control should be achieved and then your son or daughter can begin to manipulate his diabetes to suit his social life. But, even then, regularly changing the dose should not become the norm, otherwise the diabetes will become out of control again.

Changing doses when necessary can be a matter of trial and error, but this is where blood testing provides vital information. If the youngster wanted to go out to eat but was unsure how much extra insulin he should have, then he could test his blood glucose *before* the meal and decide how much insulin he should take above or below his usual dose. Testing *after* the meal for high or low levels will tell him if he had judged the amount correctly and, if not, he would have a better idea of how much to take next time. Testing before exercising is also a good idea, to allow him to expend the maximum amount of energy with no ill-effects.

Injection Devices
Syringes

Syringes are small, handy and made from disposable plastic. They are available in different sizes on prescription from your GP. The BDA recommends that each one can be used five times or until the needle becomes blunt. There is no need to swab the skin or clean the needle after use – just replace the cap and keep it with the insulin.

Syringes take all types of insulin and are the only device that can be used when insulin is free-mixed.

It's easy to see why, for some teenagers, taking a bottle of insulin and a syringe out with them is a hassle. Either it's too much to remember or they may consider that there is a stigma attached to having diabetes and using a syringe just emphasizes this. They may feel they cannot inject discreetly, even in front of friends, as syringes tend to be associated with drug addiction. Many people with diabetes sneak off to the toilet to inject if they are out, but they often feel this is unfair and unhygienic. Luckily, there is an alternative, which is extremely popular and was welcomed with open arms when it first appeared on the scene just over ten years ago – the pen.

Pens

As the name suggests, these look like cartridge pens. They are made of hardened plastic, some are fashionably colourful and look more like a fun stationery gadget than a clinical implement; there is even one due to appear on the market that is modelled on the famous Mont Blanc pen design.

The 'ink' is the cartridge of insulin and the 'nib' is the needle. When the insulin runs out, it is simply replaced by another cartridge. Likewise the needle – when it becomes blunt, another is easily attached. In fact, some pens are now completely disposable and they contain a fixed amount of insulin. When this is finished, the whole device is thrown away. However, for those who are environmentally aware, there are certain pens available that can be recycled.

If you would like more information about these, speak to your diabetes nurse. Also, if your son or daughter has a needle phobia and really cannot bear to see the needle go in, there is also a pen device that actually hides the needle. The end of this device is placed next to the skin and, with the press of a button, the needle goes in unseen and the insulin is automatically delivered. However, this kind of pen is not available on prescription – it has to be purchased.

The type of pen your teenager uses will depend on the insulin prescribed and, as the insulin comes in cartridge form, it cannot be free-mixed. However, so many mixtures are available that there's invariably something to suit everyone. Unfortunately, at the time of writing, the needles for pens (disposable or otherwise) are not available on prescription and you have to buy them. The BDA is lobbying the Government to reverse this situation.

Whether using syringes or a pen, your teenager must be given expert instruction by the diabetes specialist nurse on how to use them. Even if your son or daughter is a die-hard pen user, it is still a good idea to learn how to use a syringe in case of emergency, say if a pen is lost or broken.

Pumps

These are seldom used now (see Chapter 11) and are not manu-factured in the UK any more.

The insulin infusion pump is a small device worn on a belt or carried over the shoulder. The pump contains insulin, which is pumped through a fine plastic tube into the body via a small needle that, usually, is inserted into the stomach. The pump pro-vides a steady flow of insulin and, at mealtimes, the wearer presses a button on the pump to deliver more insulin.

The disadvantages of them are that the needle can become dis-lodged and then no insulin is delivered, which can be particularly dangerous, and they have to be worn constantly.

Jet Sprays

These gadgets deliver insulin through the skin by means of press-ure. There are no needles, but this does not mean they are pain-less. They are also very expensive to buy and, apparently, not very popular as an alternative to syringes and pens.

Human Insulin v. Animal Insulin

There's been a certain amount of controversy regarding human insulin. Human insulin is man-made and chemically identical to the insulin found in the human pancreas. It is a synthetic product made from bacteria and cannot cause AIDS or any other infectious condition. It is manufactured under sterile conditions.

Before human insulin became available in 1984, people with diabetes used insulin extracted from the pancreas of pigs or cattle and there is a slight difference between animal and human insulin. Some people who have changed from animal to human insulin have reported that their hypo symptoms have changed or have been lost, sometimes with distressing results, but so far there's no concrete scientific evidence as to why this should happen. If control of the diabetes has tightened up, then the change from a normal blood glucose to a hypo can certainly happen more quickly. The BDA has set up a working party to look into the facts, but it must be stressed that the number of people experiencing this is very small and, as your son or daughter will probably have been given human insulin right from the time their diabetes was diagnosed, they will not have experienced the changeover from animal to human insulin and so will not be affected. The BDA reports that about 8 out of 10 people with diabetes now use human insulin. Animal insulin is still available, but not for use in pen devices.

Monitoring Blood Glucose Levels

Ask most teenagers with diabetes and they will admit that testing their blood glucose levels at home or when out and about is a real bore; they feel it interferes with their lives. They think that testing is unimportant. They reckon that if they do not inject insulin, they will eventually feel unwell and so know something is wrong. Blood testing just does not seem to have the motivating influence of insulin – and this is borne out by the comments we have received from many teenagers taking part in our interviews. As Simon told us:

I do not test my blood sugars – it's not a matter of life or death. Anyway, I feel all right . . .

Yet, he would not dream of missing his insulin and takes the same dose day in, day out, no matter what he eats or what exercise he takes. It's very hit and miss but he feels 'all right'. Some people do feel quite well with high blood glucose, but it may cause damage over the years.

Testing

We talked earlier about the levels to aim for (4 to 7 mmol/l before food and 7 to 10 mmol/l about an hour after food) and these can only be accurately known by testing blood rather than the old-fashioned method of testing urine. Urine tests are still used by some people with diabetes, but doctors would far prefer them to switch to blood tests. The reason urine tests are far inferior is because they cannot give an instant picture of what's going on. The point at which the sugar in the bloodstream passes from the blood into the kidneys and is passed out in the urine is called the 'renal threshold'. Generally, the renal threshold is around 10 mmol/l, but this can vary. Some people with diabetes show the overspill of glucose in their urine at 4 mmol/l, some 13 mmol/l. A negative urine test, therefore, could be 4 or 9 mmol/l or more. Also, if urine has been in the bladder for some time, perhaps two hours or so, the result will only reflect what happened two hours ago, not what is happening at the present time, which is what home blood testing does. The information blood testing provides is easy to interpret and can be acted on immediately to the benefit of the person who needs it most – the one with diabetes.

To test blood glucose, a drop of blood is obtained from the end of the finger on the side – some people even use their ear lobes. However, using the toes is not recommended as there may be a risk of infection – if not now, then maybe in the future. Enough blood needs to be obtained to cover a pad on a test strip. There are a number of brands of these and the diabetes specialist nurse will advise and demonstrate which to use. The test strip can either be colour matched to a chart on the side of its container or be inserted into a small electronic meter, which will give a computerized reading of the result. Naturally, blood glucose meters are popular among teenagers as they are easy to carry – some are as small as a credit card or pen – and they are far quicker than taking a visual reading. It is vital that they are used according to the manufacturer's instructions, though, otherwise false readings may occur. It's best to be shown how to use the preferred meter by the diabetes specialist or GP practice nurse. Although relatively inexpensive for the job they do, these meters are a luxury, not a necessity, so don't think you *have* to buy one (though a meter might just tip the balance between whether your child actually tests his blood or not).

Your son or daughter will be told, ideally, how often they should perform tests and asked to record the results in a special diary or logbook. Recording results is something teenagers are not too keen on either. Eddie, 18, says:

I'm not very scientific about keeping records of my blood tests – I do two or more a day but hardly ever get around to writing them down.

Well, at least he's doing them – most teenagers manage to reach a compromise between how many tests the clinic suggests and how many they think they should do.

Long-term Blood Tests

Home blood test results are useful to the doctor in the clinic, but the results of long-term blood tests can provide further information. They are particularly useful if the teenager forgets his book, writes down false results (another little foible!) or the doctor wants to compare laboratory results with the home results. Long-term blood tests are also another method of checking how effectively the diabetes is being controlled.

The diabetes clinic will either perform a glycosylated haemoglobin (HbA1C) or a fructosamine test. The HbA1C shows the average blood glucose level over the last six to eight weeks, while the fructosamine test shows what it has been over the previous two to three weeks. What is considered a normal result can vary from hospital to hospital, so an explanation of the results is necessary.

These tests are extremely valuable as the day-to-day variations of home blood testing can't give the broad picture that the HbA1C, in particular, provides. However, interpreting and acting on home results are key to a good HbA1C or fructosamine result, which, in turn, paves the way to good health in the future. In Chapter 4, we explore the problems that can occur if there is a refusal to test or false results are given.

It does seem that blood testing at home commonly causes teenagers to become fed up and many parents worry that they're not exactly doing their utmost to keep tabs on their control. Liz – mother of 14-year-old Amy – says:

She handles her diabetes well but does hate taking her blood, which causes friction at times. I worry about this but am afraid of putting too much pressure on her and making her feel worse about her diabetes. My one great wish is for better blood testing equipment – less obtrusive. When are they going to produce the infra-red blood tester we've heard about?

The answer to that is, in the (hopefully) not too distant future. The idea is that infra-red readings could be taken from a compact tester worn on the wrist. Presumably, it would look similar to the heart/pulse rate monitors now – neat, unobtrusive, no needle required and with a continuous read-out of data. Perfect! Anyone who has diabetes would welcome this gadget, so our message to the companies involved in developing infra-red testing equipment is – the sooner the better, please! (See Chapter 11).

Chapter 4

HYPERS AND HYPOS – COPING WITH THE HIGHS AND LOWS

Trying to control blood glucose levels is not always easy, particularly for the adolescent. Life is complicated enough with all the physical and mental changes taking place and diabetes creates even more problems. Testing blood glucose becomes a hassle that is made worse in the teenager's mind because the doctors and nurses at the clinic seem so fixated with 'numbers'. There is, of course, a good reason for the medical professionals' concern. They want your son or daughter to stay healthy while being able to lead as normal a life as possible. They are concerned that poor control can lead to problems which can disrupt a teenager's lifestyle. Low blood glucose levels can cause hypos, which are certainly disruptive, while running high glucose levels can increase the risk of developing the complications of diabetes in the future.

Complications of Diabetes – the Facts

The possible complications of diabetes are real and cannot be ignored. It's natural for many teenagers (and parents) to try and put their fears to the back of their mind, telling themselves that it simply won't happen to them. Indeed, research has found that 25 per cent of insulin-dependent diabetics do *not* develop the complications of diabetes and if a person with diabetes does not develop complications after 25 years of having the condition, then the chances of their suffering from them in the future are slim. It is not known why some people with diabetes develop complications and others appear to be immune; researchers feel this is probably due to their genetic make-up.

What Are the Complications?

The complications of diabetes are indigenous to people who have had diabetes for many years and are not seen in people who do not have the condition.

Diabetic Retinopathy

This is damage to the retina at the back of the eye, caused by restricted blood flow or bleeding into the back of the eye from abnormal blood vessels.

It can be diagnosed by looking into the eye with an opthalmoscope, and this is something that will be checked regularly. Some clinics have the equipment to take pictures of the eye, but, even if they do not, your son or daughter should have their eyes checked by a skilled doctor. If retinopathy is discovered, he or she will be referred to an opthalmologist. If necessary, the condition can be slowed down or stopped by the use of laser therapy, which seals the abnormal blood vessels.

Your son or daughter will not be able to tell if there is any damage as this can only be seen when a trained person gives them a proper examination, which is why regular checks are vital. If he or she starts to experience loss of vision, then urgent treatment is necessary as diabetic retinopathy can lead to blindness. Fortunately, this happens in only a small number of people, but it is crucial that examinations are carried out at least once a year to detect any changes, which your child would not notice.

Diabetic Nephropathy

This means damage to the kidneys. At every clinic check-up, your son or daughter will be given a urine test and part of this test shows whether protein is present in the urine – one way of detecting kidney damage. The more protein is found, the greater the damage to the kidneys. Blood tests will verify what's going on.

Checks will also be made on blood pressure as it's known that keeping the blood pressure normal slows down the progression of kidney failure, and this can be helped by medication.

Diabetic Neuropathy

This is damage to the nerves, particularly in the legs, which leads to lack of, or complete loss of, feeling. When it occurs, it can be dangerous as then an injury to the foot or leg might not be felt and could become infected. Taking this scenario to its worst extreme, gangrene could set in, necessitating amputation. Anna has had diabetes for 30 years and was admitted to hospital with a broken ankle:

> *I fell in the street . . . when I tried to get up, I couldn't move. My ankle was swelling up, but I couldn't feel anything. I was amazed when my ankle was X-rayed and I was told it was broken . . . I couldn't believe it.*

Your teenager should be told how important it is to take care of their feet so that no infections occur, and verrucas, bunions and so on should be expertly treated by a chiropodist. Neuropathy is not always painless – some people with diabetes describe a burning sensation in their legs and feet – but this can be improved by good control. The clinic and the BDA can both provide plenty of information on how best to look after the feet.

Nerve damage can also occur in the internal organs, like the bladder and bowel, and can cause impotence.

People with diabetes are also more prone to problems with the circulation, which can lead to heart disease, foot and leg ulcers and gangrene. However, circulatory problems are not specifically complications of diabetes as they are also seen in those without it.

Lessening the Risk

So, how can these complications be prevented? Essentially, they occur after years of poorly controlled diabetes. The Diabetes Control and Complications Trial, a study in the United States, the results of which were published in September 1993, took 1,400 people with insulin-dependent diabetes and divided them into two groups. The group with good control (their HbA1C results averaging 7.2 per cent) had 60 per cent less retinopathy, nephropathy and neuropathy than the second group with poorer control. However, this group had four injections a day or a continuous infusion pump, and the down side was that there was an increase in the number of hypos that participants had in order to control their diabetes as tightly as possible. Some of the patients had full-blown hypos – that is, they reached the stage where they needed assistance from someone else. This group also had unparalleled support from many healthcare professionals, but this was part of the trial and not a normal way of life.

The trial showed that there is no doubt that good control reduces the complications of diabetes, but it also showed that *achieving* constant good control is not easy. You have to face facts: your child will not have the constant support of an army of doctors, nurses, dieticians and psychologists that the guinea pigs in the trial did. To gain tight control, she will have to discipline herself assiduously, and such control may result in more hypos (although these will not necessarily be severe if she is fully aware of early warning signs and acts immediately any of these occur). Hypos – unless they are severe and frequent – do not cause lasting damage, except perhaps to self-confidence.

As we advised in the previous chapter, perhaps a good compromise is to aim for glucose levels of between 4 and 10 mmol/l (the higher figure after meals) rather than to strive for one of between 3.5 and 8 mmol/l (apart from in pregnancy). Yet, as we noted, despite being told that good control is important to prevent the complications of diabetes, blood tests still remain an area of conflict in many homes.

So, if your son or daughter refuses to test, what can you do about it? If the subject of testing becomes a constant battle, in the short term, only you will be the loser. Unfortunately, in the long term your child could be the one to lose. But, however anxious you feel about this, don't use complications as a threat or a weapon, for instilling fear may have the opposite effect and the teenager may irrationally reason, 'If I don't test then I won't have to know what's going on so that's fine by me'.

She may even make up results just to stop you going on about it. Teenagers (and adults) often present beautifully kept log books to the doctor, full of seemingly perfect results, which are mainly false. Those who are a dab hand at deception will put in the odd high or low sugar to add a touch of realism (although, in fairness, there are those who keep genuinely tidy log books and record honest results). Yet, it's a fact that tidiness is not a common trait among teenagers and the majority of log books reflect this, so a pristine log book inevitably arouses suspicion. A high HbA1C will reflect just how accurate the home blood test results actually are!

Keep calm when faced with a non-testing teenager. Try to explain gently that good control will enable her to get the best out of life. Knowing her blood glucose levels means that she can adjust insulin or food depending on her activity, and that knowing her glucose levels and being able to act on them will prevent any social embarrassments, like unexpected hypos or comments about how many times she visits the toilet in an evening and how much she's drinking (symptoms of high glucose). Remind her that she is doing this for herself and her future.

Perhaps you could reach a compromise about when tests are done. If you can both agree on a routine, this may help. For example:

- Monday, test before breakfast
- Tuesday, test before lunch (if this is difficult for some reason, then pick another time, such as when she gets home from school)
- Wednesday, before dinner
  and so on through the week.

Alternatively, she could choose two days during the week on which she could test three or four times.

If you still find you are not winning, then speak to your young-ster's diabetes specialist nurse as she may find it easier to relate to her. Quite often, a teenager will test to please the nurse because she doesn't want to let her down. Psychologically, someone who cares and understands the situation but is not emotionally involved as such can work wonders.

Hypers – Warning Signs of High Blood Glucose Levels

The most common symptoms of high blood glucose (hyper-glycaemia) do not occur until the blood glucose level rises above about 14 mmol/l. Therefore, your child may feel perfectly well even if her blood glucose is high. It is quite common for a person with diabetes to get used to high sugar levels and when they come down to *normal*, they feel like they're having a hypo. The more common symptoms of hyperglycaemia are:

- passing more urine and making frequent trips to the toilet, noticeably at night
- excessive thirst
- lethargy, falling asleep at unusual times
- weight loss.

You may notice your son or daughters' mouth is dry and cracks develop at the corners of the mouth. He or she may develop thrush around the genitals (although this may not be mentioned). You may notice that he or she complains of blurred vision, holds a book at an unusual distance or may not seem to be able to focus on the television (the blurred vision is caused by the lens of the eye becoming full of sugar, distorting the vision). There may be a lack of concentration, with school work suffering. If she were to test her blood glucose she would find it high most of the time. Levels over 10 mmol/l means her diabetes is out of control, but if she has the symptoms we've described, then her blood glucose must be constantly over 15 mmol/l.

When blood glucose levels are very high through neglect or illness, ketones may be found in the urine (see later in this chapter). If she develops ketones, she will progress to having the symptoms listed later in this chapter. Vomiting should always be taken seriously as this can lead to ketoacidosis, or diabetic coma. If your child vomits twice or more, contact your diabetes clinic immediately or go to the nearest hospital casualty department.

If your teenager is not showing obvious signs of being ill, but you have spotted some of the symptoms mentioned above, then you may have to use a little cunning to actually get her to admit that she does, in fact, feel unwell. You could try mentioning that she looks rather under the weather and casually asking what her blood glucose is doing. Ask her (casually again) if it's time she saw the diabetes specialist nurse. Try not to get into an argument; use the softly softly approach.

Hypers can be caused by not taking enough insulin. Sue told us:

I was meant to be on two injections a day. I hated having diabetes so I would only take one injection in the morning, even though I assured mum I had done the other one at night. I couldn't stand the constant nagging . . . I didn't feel very well but I got used to feeling thirsty . . . in the end the clinic discovered I had constantly high glucose levels as the blood test results I'd made up didn't come anywhere near the result of the HbA1C. I was referred to a psychologist who helped me sort things out.

David's story was similar:

My doctor put me on four injections a day, even though I'd told him I didn't want to go up from two. I stopped taking the lunchtime injection at school. It was embarrassing as I had to go to the secretary's office to do my injection. In the end, I just didn't bother. No one knew until my long-term blood test results came through . . .

If you feel your teenager may be missing out injections, then you may have to be subtly vigilant. How quickly do they get through their store of insulin? It's easy to work out how often a cartridge in a pen needs to be changed: there are 150 units in a normal cartridge and 300 units in the disposable pens, so you can tell how much insulin she *needs* compared to how much she seems to be *using* from the 'store' in the fridge. If she seems to take a long time to get through a week's supply, then ask her to be honest with you – is she missing out some injections?

In David's case, the reason he had been changed to four injections should have been thoroughly explained by his doctor so that he could clearly see the advantages, but he should not have been bludgeoned into it. Most teenagers come around to the multiple injection regime happily when they really see the benefits – but that can take time. As for Sue, she resented having diabetes and injecting only reminded her of the predicament, so she did the bare minimum. Counselling encouraged her to talk over her feelings and finally come to terms with the situation, accepting that doing more injections would make her life better. Always remind your child that you care, and support and encourage her when blood test results are good and she is coping well. Rebelling is quite normal and we discuss this further in Chapter 9.

Another obvious cause of hyperglycaemia is eating sweets as if there's no tomorrow or shunning diet drinks in favour of regular colas and so on. This problem is covered in Chapter 6 on diet.

Illness

Illness and, in particular, any type of infection can cause a rise in blood glucose levels (although this does not always happen). It is vital that your child continues to take insulin, even if she is off food. *Never stop insulin.*

During periods of illness, your son or daughter may require more insulin than usual, so blood glucose should be checked regularly – at least every two hours. Extra doses of short-acting insulin should be taken if blood tests are high. Also, test urine for ketones and contact your diabetes nurse or doctor if symptoms persist or even if there are no ketones but she vomits twice or more.

If your son or daughter has no appetite, then give sugary drinks to maintain the carbohydrate and fluid intake. A glass of Lucozade, fruit juice or ordinary non-diet cola should be given hourly. If even fluids cannot be tolerated, then the youngster should be in hospital. However, don't worry every time the teenager has a cold – these do not necessarily cause any rise in blood glucose levels. Ordinary medicines have only a tiny sugar content so will not be the cause of high glucose levels if she uses them, but there are plenty of sugar-free alternatives if preferred.

Suggested Food and Drink When Unwell
Each of the following contains 10 g (¼ oz) of carbohydrate.

- 50 ml (2 fl oz) of Lucozade
- 100 ml (4 fl oz) non-diet cola
- 200 ml (7 fl oz) milk
- 100 ml (4 fl oz) fruit juice
- 50 g (2 oz) ice-cream
- 50 g (2 oz) non-diet yoghurt (half a small pot)
- 1 small banana
- 1 pear, orange or apple
- 2 level teaspoons/2 lumps of sugar or honey
- 3 glucose tablets.

Ketones
When blood glucose levels are very high, through neglect or during periods of illness, ketones can be found in the urine. As we mentioned earlier in this book, this occurs when the body breaks down fat to make energy as there is not enough insulin to convert sugar into energy.

A build-up of ketones is dangerous as these are a poisonous acid that can eventually lead to ketoacidosis, or diabetic coma. As well as high blood glucose, symptoms to look out for are:

- weight loss

- nausea
- vomiting
- stomach cramps
- breath smelling of acetone or pear drops
- shallow breathing.

Ketoacidosis must be treated urgently as it can result in coma and eventually death. If you recognize the recurrence of any of the symptoms your son or daughter had before being diagnosed as having diabetes, you must act and test for ketones. This is just a matter of wetting the pad of a ketone strip (available on prescription) in urine, timing and matching the pad against the colours on the side of the bottle. You should also insist on a test if there is illness or vomiting.

Stressful Situations

Stress is also a cause of high blood glucose levels, but there is not much one can do about this if the event or worry causing the stress is over quickly. However, exams are a common cause of anxiety and the preparation for and sitting of these can go on for weeks, often causing genuine problems with control. Richard reports:

Just before my exams, I felt very tired and often had to get up during the night to go to the toilet. Once they were underway, I was very embarrassed to have to be accompanied to the loo by a teacher during the GCSE maths exam. I'll admit I was so engrossed in my GCSEs, I didn't bother testing my sugars. My mum noticed I was thirsty and made me test. I was shocked when I found my blood glucose was 20 and staying there. I spoke to my diabetes nurse and she suggested I increase my insulin while the exams were on. When it came to my 'A' levels, I increased my insulin by half the normal dose again and felt far better.

If the teenager is going through a stressful time, she will probably put diabetes on the back burner. As well as forgetting to test, she may forget to eat, which could cause problems with hypos. It's even more important than usual to test when there's a change in the day-to-day routine as it is easy to lose control when glucose levels are allowed to fluctuate.

But, some forms of stress may be less obvious. Samantha hated PE, particularly hockey:

> *I suppose it stemmed from the time I had a hypo on the field. I had forgotten to eat my snack, but I did have some glucose tablets in my tracksuit pocket and knew what to do. When she saw me eating my glucose, the PE teacher went into a real panic. She made me sit out for the rest of the lesson, even though I then ate my snack and was perfectly able to carry on. After that, she asked at every lesson whether I'd had my snack and if I was OK – always in front of my friends. It was so embarrassing.*

Samantha noticed that her glucose levels seemed to rise a couple of days before PE but went back to normal the day after and she knew hockey was the culprit! Eventually, Sam told her diabetes nurse, who visited the school and had a word with the PE teacher. It turned out that the teacher was petrified Sam would collapse without warning during a lesson. The nurse explained that Sam knew her warning signs and what to do. The teacher took a low-key approach to the matter after this, Sam felt less hassled and her glucose levels settled down.

If your youngster's glucose levels rise at certain times of the day or week and there's no obvious reason for it (say, dietary), then try to talk through whether or not something is bothering her – it could well be something she's got herself into a state over which could be sorted out simply and with no fuss.

Other Reasons For High Glucose Levels

These include the following:

- high glucose following a hypo (see section on hypos below)

46

- periods (these can cause high or low glucose levels, see Chapter 2)
- pregnancy – the reason for this is hormonal (see Chapter 8).

Hypos – What to Do

A hypo is the commonly used short form of the term hypoglycaemia, which is low blood glucose. A hypo occurs when the blood glucose level falls below 3 mmol/l, but many people with diabetes have warning signs before their glucose levels become this low and are usually able to recognize their own symptoms of an impending hypo.

The most common symptoms are sweating, trembling, feeling dizzy. Some people have blurred vision (which can be confused with high blood glucose), while some say they feel a kind of numbness, like pins and needles, around the mouth. They may have a change in personality – some become aggressive, some just go very pale and quiet. The symptoms of a hypo should be treated immediately by eating or drinking something sugary (such as non-diet cola or Lucozade, three glucose tablets or some chocolate). If the youngster does not feel better within a few minutes, then she should have some more. Once she feels better, she should have some form of starchy carbohydrate, such as a small sandwich, to maintain the glucose levels, as the effects of sugary foods do not last long.

Your child should *always* carry some form of sugar with her in case of hypos. Don't let her make excuses, such as, 'I can always go to a sweet shop', as that's not good enough – a hypo can happen anywhere, and there are no sweet shops when you are stuck in a traffic jam or cycling down a country lane!

It is necessary to take action immediately because if warning signs are ignored and the hypo becomes too advanced, then she may be unable to take food or drink by mouth. She may become aggressive, confused or even unconscious – some people can even 'fit'. If she is aggressive, never shout at her as this often makes things worse. She will eventually quieten down and become difficult to rouse. At this point, you could try rubbing jam or honey on to her gums and inside the cheeks – be careful not to be bitten! Alternatively, you could use a special glucose gel called Hypostop, which has a long nozzle and can be squirted directly into the side of the mouth. Massage the cheek from the outside. The bottle is marked so you will know how much to give. Either way, the sugary substance will be absorbed through the cheek lining or swallowed with the saliva. Incidentally, glucose gel tastes rather nasty and she may spit it out so always err on the safe side and give plenty.

A hypo can be a frightening experience for everyone concerned, particularly if your teenager becomes unconscious. If she does go into a fit, do not attempt to give anything by mouth except Hypostop. Turn her on to her side and move away any objects on which she may hurt herself.

If glucose gel does not work, give an injection of glucagon (see below). If you are unable to bring her round in 20 minutes (which is pretty unlikely), then call an ambulance. The paramedics will give glucose intravenously. You should also call an ambulance if you cannot bring your child round with glucose gel and do not have any glucagon in the house.

Glucagon

This is a hormone that works in the opposite way to insulin. It causes the liver to release its own supply of glucose should the level in the blood become too low.

A glucagon injection comes in kit form and you can get this on prescription from your GP. The kit consists of a syringe and two small bottles (one contains a powder, the other sterile water to mix with it). Read the instructions and become familiar with the equipment in case you need to use it. Your diabetes nurse may be able to let you have a practise run at drawing up as it can be tricky, especially with shaking hands! Note, however, that, at the time of writing, the kit has just been changed. The new kit is called GlucaGen and the water is already drawn up in the syringe.

Glucagon should be injected into the upper arm, the thigh or the top outer quarter of the buttock. The child should come round within 10 to 20 minutes of receiving the injection. She may be sick, but this is not unusual following an injection of glucagon.

Once she has recovered, give a sweet drink, followed by starchy food – little and often. However, if you are really worried, do not feel you have to cope just because you have the equipment – call an ambulance instead. Parents are often concerned that hypos may cause brain damage in their child, but this is not the case so long as severe hypos do not occur frequently. The long-term risks of high blood glucose levels are far more dangerous than the occasional hypo.

Night Hypos and Rebound Hyperglycaemia

Many parents of children who have diabetes are very frightened of night hypos. They fear that the child could die, but this is not true. In the majority of cases, the child wakes up because she actually feels the hypo coming on. If she doesn't, the body's own supply of the hormone glucagon rises and this, in turn, causes a release of sugar, which is stored in the liver. The result of this is a rise in the blood glucose level and she comes out of her hypo. Indeed, high glucose levels in the morning could indicate that a hypo occurred during the night (rebound hyperglycaemia). *Never* give extra insulin to bring down the sugar level as this is likely to cause another hypo later on. Instead, try to work out why it happened. Was the bedtime snack forgotten? Did she take more than her usual dose of insulin? Did she exercise more than normal during the day or in the evening (hypos can be delayed, coming on up to 12 hours after strenuous exercise)? If there does not seem to be a reason for the high level and neither of you can fathom it out, then the only way to get an answer is to test the blood glucose at around 2 a.m. for a few nights. If the level is low at that time, then the evening dose of medium-acting insulin will need to be decreased.

Alcohol

One area of real danger with hypos can be when drinking alcohol. There is no reason for people with diabetes to become teetotal, but they should be aware of the potential problems. As we explained above, the liver stores glucose, which can be released into the bloodstream should a hypo occur. However, alcohol *blocks* that mechanism and can result in more severe – and potentially dangerous – hypoglycaemia. The higher the alcohol content of the drink, the more likely the mechanism is to be blocked.

Some lagers are marketed as low in sugar, but they should be avoided by those with diabetes as they often have a high alcohol content. It is actually safer to drink ordinary lager. Spirits are relatively low in calories, but the high alcohol content should be taken into consideration. Initially, alcohol can cause the blood glucose level to rise, but it may well fall later on. When your son or daughter (quite naturally) doesn't want to be left out of having a drink with friends, then he or she should know the following rules to do so safely:

- never drink on an empty stomach – have a meal with plenty of starchy carbohydrate (such as a pizza) beforehand
- have a substantial starchy snack at bedtime (such as cereal) to prevent a hypo during the night, when too much alcohol and not enough food could have very dangerous effects (as the release of glucose from the liver may be blocked by the alcohol)

See Chapter 8 for more about social drinking, partying, dances and so on.

The Causes of Hypos

Hypos can be caused by any of the following:

- Too much insulin. It's not unknown for people with diabetes to muddle the dose up from time to time. If this has happened, test blood glucose regularly and advise her to eat some extra carbohydrate. If the teenager is unsure as to whether or not she has actually given herself the injection at all, assume she has. She should *not* have more insulin, just take the next dose when it's due.

- Extra exercise.
- Excess alcohol.
- Missed or delayed meals. Eating regularly should prevent hypoglycaemia, but, by their very nature, teenagers tend not to eat regularly – especially if they are at work rather than school. See Chapter 6 for suggestions on diet.
- Not reducing insulin enough when changing to a new injection site from a lumpy one.
- Early pregnancy.
- Periods.

The Fear of Hypos

Many teenagers (and parents) develop a fear of hypos, often through hearing horror stories or having had a bad experience. Sonia – now 18 – told us:

My fear of hypos stemmed from my mother. When I was nine, I had a bad hypo during the night and ended up in hospital. I can't remember much about it now but for years afterwards, my mother would make me eat an enormous bedtime snack, saying, 'You don't want another hypo like the one that put you in hospital'. Eventually, I became so paranoid about hypos I ran my sugars high to avoid them. This was becoming a real problem and I ended up seeing a psychologist about my fear. It's been hard to overcome this fear, but now I know that I'm not going to keel over the minute my sugars are low; I trust my warning signs and take action immediately.

When the fear of hypos prevents diabetes from being well-controlled, there is certainly a problem. As a parent, you want to see your child fit and well. A hypo can unnerve you and make you anxious, even if it is mild. However, if she is not even having the occasional *mild* hypo, then her glucose levels must be pretty high and that's a real worry, because then there is a risk of long-term problems.

Of course, severe hypoglycaemia is a problem. This should be discussed at the diabetes clinic and a solution found by adjusting insulin or diet. If anxiety is causing your son or daughter to run her glucose levels high, then talk this over with her doctor or diabetes nurse. They may refer your teenager to a psychologist and this will be your best bet if they or you are unable to reassure the teenager (or yourself) that a solution can be found.

Chapter 5

'I DON'T WANT TO BE DIFFERENT!'

Few young teenagers want to stand out from their peers. Each group of friends has its own dress code, musical and social preferences. It's really not until later adolescence that young people have the confidence to break free and be completely individual. So, surely it follows that a boy or girl with diabetes resents having to be 'different' – or does it?

Naturally, nobody who has diabetes would *choose* to have it, yet many of the comments we received suggested that this 'difference' could be used to positive effect:

It's part of me, it's my own thing.

I stopped thinking of myself as 'different' because I haven't missed out on anything that I've wanted to do because of my diabetes. I would say that it's made me do more.

I have no qualms at all about injecting in front of my friends. People are, by nature, inquisitive, so I try and answer all their questions . . . it makes a good starting point for new relationships.

A few comments did give us cause for concern, however. For instance, John – now 24 – felt his experiences had been pretty negative:

. . . being scared to tell people you have diabetes because sticking needles in one's arms isn't the said thing to do . . . Most people haven't a clue about it and don't want to know either. It's a very awkward and embarrassing thing to teach people about diabetes.

Yet, this was by no means the majority opinion, leading us to speculate how John's diabetes had been handled when he was first diagnosed, at the age of 15. Poor handling, either by the medical team or by overreactive parents who, with the best will in the world, makes a child feel apart from 'normality', perhaps because of overcossetting them and being unwilling to 'let go'.

Most of the teenagers we interviewed were relaxed about doing whatever they had to do in front of their friends:

My friends think it's cool that I can eat in class, get into early dinners and they think I'm brave injecting. Everyone tests their blood and two of my friends have each voluntarily stuck empty needles in themselves to see what I go through.

It has brought my friends a lot closer to me. They are genuinely interested and I enjoy explaining it to them.

They know it must be a hassle, but then so is doing homework.

My friends often want to do my injections for me when I'm at school. Their support is great and they have also learned something.

But Gemma, 15, voices the understandable anxieties of someone with diabetes:

You're constantly worrying about going hypo, doing injections on time, eating enough. I was petrified I'd go hypo when I went caving and rock-climbing; there was no way I'd be able to get at my Hypostop without endangering my life. I was OK, though, and you have to grit your teeth when you feel like that, otherwise you'd never do anything.

It's true that having diabetes makes you different, but many gritty youngsters show how this can be turned to their advantage. Jill, now 18, admitted that she felt different because of her diabetes, but decided to go the whole hog and be *completely* different from the crowd:

> *I dyed my hair all sorts of colours, I loved dressing really outrageously. I refused to wear Doc Martens just because everyone else did. I loved all the attention. I've settled down a lot now and, to be honest, I'm finding life a bit boring.*

Claire says:

> *I felt myself going hypo when I was with this boyfriend and he fed me dextrose in a very romantic way. It was different, that's for sure!*

Jeremy admits:

> *I like being different without actually being conspicuous. Sometimes it's a novelty to be different. Diabetes is not a disability and I've got the same chances as everyone else.*

Tim disagreed:

> *I don't like being different in this way at all. I can't see anything good about having to think ahead and plan when everyone else just does what they want. I don't go out much, it's too much of a hassle and I don't want to be labelled 'different', thank you very much.*

If your newly diagnosed teenager is worried about being 'different', then the best help you can give is to encourage him to carry on with life as it was before and to talk openly, sharing his feelings with others. He must not be made to feel that there is anything taboo about diabetes or anything to be ashamed of. Injecting may well be associated with junkies, but assure him that he is not taking drugs of any kind – insulin is a hormone, not a drug as such.

If he resents the total dependence he knows he must now have on insulin, you can help him realize that all of us are dependent on something or someone in one way or another right through our lives. Fussing, treating your teenager as a semi-invalid, pandering to his slightest whim and nagging him constantly about injections, blood tests and food will only build up problems for the future. Don't use bribery, offering prizes of one sort or another for doing blood tests and so on – he'll have you over a barrel in no time, and you'll soon run out of money! Overlooking bad behaviour because he has diabetes is also quite the wrong approach. Brothers, sisters and friends will soon be envious at what he gets away with. Then, your child will be singled out as different, but in a completely negative way.

However, there are certain concessions you can make. If the hospital has provided him with syringes and he really does feel this will be associated with drugs, then move heaven and earth to get him a pen device – his diabetes specialist nurse is sure to help. Bona fide needle-phobics could try the pen device with the concealed needle that we mentioned in Chapter 3 and maybe consider having some counselling (the clinic may recommend a psychologist if needle-phobia really is the case).

Carrying identity may be a bone of contention for some teenagers, but this really is a must in case they become hypo or hyper when they are out and about. Specialist jewellery is recognized worldwide, but don't waste time arguing the pros and cons of identity cards or jewellery that they think look unfashionable (although there is a range of medallions available depicting favourite sports, which might appeal, as well as fashionable-looking bracelets, some of which contain a central emergency number for those who subscribe to have their medical details stored on computer). Why not suggest trendy army ID tags (available from surplus stores) or dog tags (look in the classified section of pet magazines, many of which advertise tags shaped like bones, hearts or the more usual round shape). Any of these can have a simple inscription added, such as 'diabetic on insulin', a name and phone number. Hopefully, these might appeal to the fashion-conscious side of their nature!

If your son or daughter makes a fuss about carrying glucose

tablets and/or equipment, then point out that they always seem to have a pocket or a rucksack and that carrying a personal stereo around never seemed to present problems before, so why should this? Unfortunately, at the time of writing, the ideal solution of bumbags seem to have gone out of fashion (except for sport). But there are alternatives, such as jacket pockets, a sports bag or even hidden belts that are worn under clothes (travellers often use hidden belts for keeping their money safe while abroad and these are available from most luggage shops or department stores). Don't expect your teenager to buy anything like this for himself, but it's hardly bribery and corruption if you provide the money for a belt, bag or whatever.

Sleeping Habits

It's a rare teenager who doesn't spend weekends and holidays going to bed late and getting up hours after the rest of the household the following morning. You may find yourself becoming anxious that the slumbering heap in the bed upstairs should be having his morning insulin at a time the rest of the world calls breakfast. Should he be woken, leading to a row along the lines of, 'Now I have diabetes I can't even sleep in!'? Relax, the lie-ins can continue.

Sophie, 15, explains:

I'm on four pen injections a day. Occasionally I wake up really late – around lunchtime – then I usually have a large breakfast instead of lunch. I've missed the early meal and the insulin, so I only have three injections that day . . . I don't try and squeeze four injections in because it would mean eating non-stop.

Steve says:

I'm on two injections of pre-mixed insulin. When I wake up late I cut my morning insulin dose by a third, have breakfast and miss out what would have been my mid-morning snack.

As we discussed in the previous chapter, a regime of four injections a day is probably the ideal for the teenager's erratic lifestyle. Because each meal is covered by a separate dose of short-acting insulin, the timing of meals can be so much more flexible.

'Sleepover' parties can be another cause of anxiety for parents of younger teenagers with diabetes. It's the opposite problem to the long lie-in with the worries this time being will they get any sleep at all and will they eat all night? Perhaps worse, will they actually eat *anything*?

Sleepovers begin to rear their heads when children are around ten years old. Instead of just one friend staying the night, the child insists on at least half a dozen, and this inevitably ends in a sleepless night for the entire household, with bleary-eyed, irritable children (and adults!) and the compulsory midnight feast.

When children are still around primary school age, it's far easier to keep control of their social lives, simply because you are more likely to know their friend's parents and can discuss eating arrangements with them when your child goes to stay and is in their care. But, when a child goes on to secondary school, many parents find themselves increasingly cut off from playground socializing. At this stage, the child is more likely to meet children you have not previously known and they may be unaware that your son or daughter has diabetes.

When your teenager has been invited to a sleepover party, don't let anxiety make you try to stop him going – that's grounds for rebellion. Take the line that he should now be responsible for doing his injections and eating properly without having to be reminded by you or another parent, so it's up to him if he wants to go. However, if your son or daughter is under 16, then it is absolutely right that you insist on a contact number, which you should call to confirm that there will be an adult on the premises. It would be irresponsible of parents to leave a group of children (which is, after all, what they still are) alone all night, whether or not someone in the group has diabetes. When you make your phonecall, you can mention in passing that your son or daughter has diabetes and, although he or she would prefer not to have any special attention, you wanted them to know about this in case of any problems.

You will have to leave the eating arrangements to your teenager's discretion, but could suggest he takes a large bottle of diet cola, which can be pooled with the rest of the drinks. How much sleep your child gets will not affect his diabetes control, so long as he takes snacks to stop his glucose levels falling low in the night when he would normally be asleep. In Chapter 8, we talk about teenage parties in general and include information on alcohol, drugs, all-night raves and more.

Unsociable Hours

You may have found (or are about to find out) that most adolescents prefer not to be tied to set eating times when they are out and about with their friends. So, having diabetes may put your son or daughter in a difficult situation. Your daughter will not want to stop the momentum of a fruitful shopping expedition by insisting that everyone must be sitting down and ready for lunch at the pizza restaurant at one o'clock sharp and your son probably wouldn't think it cool to whip out a sandwich while he's chatting up a girl. Teenagers often go to meet friends with no set plan in mind, too – perhaps a vague, 'We're going up to town', or 'We'll decide what we're doing when we meet'. They tend to have little regard for time, spend hours making arrangements, then changing them. Of course, it would be unfair to say that *all* teenagers are like this as there are those who are well-organized and excellent time-keepers, but we, personally, don't know any.

So, if your teenager seems socially chaotic, you may well be worrying how this lifestyle is going to fit in with diabetes. The blunt answer from the boys and girls in our survey is that diabetes has to fit in with their lives, not the other way round:

You have to get on with life . . . control your diabetes, don't let it control you!

You can have a good time and enjoy yourself just like your friends. You have to stop at certain limits for health reasons . . . but then the kind of things I'm talking about, like smoking and drugs, are not good for anyone. Nor is eating junk all the time.

Obey doctor's orders, then you can do more of what you want.

Be prepared – then you can take life as it comes.

Take it easy . . . you get used to having it and you can use your knowledge of diabetes to make it fit in with your life.

This attitude – within a certain amount of reason – is endorsed by medical experts.

Essentially, finding a flexible regime that suits the teenager and controls his diabetes takes understanding and patience from both sides – the teenager and the professionals. You, as a parent, are very much pig in the middle, though, obviously, you can help and advise when necessary. But, driving yourself and your son or daughter crazy with anxiety is only going to push a wedge between you.

Living with diabetes and fitting it comfortably into a hectic lifestyle is the teenager's responsibility to himself. Providing he is well-educated in the mechanics and boundaries of the condition, there is no reason for him not to adapt his regime to suit the situation at hand. As we suggested earlier, multiple injections may sound unacceptable at first, but most teenagers quickly realize the advantages of this. Injecting short-acting insulin to cover each meal means that they can, within reason, eat when they want to and not be tied down to restricting times. Carrying the pen, ID and hypostoppers (such as glucose tablets) at all times means they are, more or less, covered for every eventuality and if a conventional lunchtime is missed, then a meal suggested at three o'clock in the afternoon, your teenager is able to be as spontaneous as his friends.

Mark, 16, says:

But there's always this little voice in my head querying whether I've had enough carbohydrate and you always need to plan ahead if you go out early on a night as you may find yourself in a situation where food is not available. There are ways around this problem, but it does restrict your enjoyment sometimes.

If your teenager complains that he feels restricted by his current regime, do your best to make him take steps to sort things out. As Suzanne, aged 17, advises:

If you don't get on top of your diabetes, it will get hold of your life like the devil and make it hell. Control your diabetes and make it work for you. These days there is so much someone with diabetes can do, whereas in the past there were many restrictions.

Peter says:

I keep my pen and my glucose tablets in my jacket pocket at all times. Once I know we're soon to eat, I inject. Sometimes I get out a piece of paper at the same time and balance it on my leg so it looks as though I'm going to write something down (with the 'pen'). I inject straight through my trousers and no one notices!

Injecting through clothes is one way round the problem of being discreet when there's no privacy. It's a good solution, although your child should be aware that injecting through clothes will blunt the needle fairly quickly.

Peer Pressure

You may find that your son or daughter is friendly with a group that you would prefer he or she did not mix with. These feelings in themselves can lead to arguments. The first thing you have to consider in such a situation is this: does this dislike/distrust of your child's friends have anything to do with you being over-protective because he has diabetes? If this is the *only* thing that bothers you, give him the benefit of the doubt. Obviously, if you suspect (or have evidence) that the group he goes around with take drugs or are delinquents, then you certainly need to have a serious discussion as to the possible repercussions of these friendships. But, surely this would apply whether he had diabetes or not? Make sure you have your facts straight first – false accusations about your child's friends are bound to lead to fireworks. However, if you simply have a nagging feeling that your teenager is up to no good just because you don't like the look of his friends, think again.

There are plenty of common misunderstandings about peer pressure, and this has been borne out by sociological studies. Your teenager may like to dress like the crowd and be seen as 'one of them', but is he really so passive that he is willing to be led like a lamb into doing things that he knows are wrong?

Most adolescents want to push the barriers to see how much they can get away with, whether that means drinking alcohol when they are under age, refusing to help in the house or bunking school. They need to find out for themselves what is acceptable, what is not acceptable and, yes, they need to rebel. They need to prove their independence and find out who they are. If you share a warm, loving relationship with your child, then that child is far less likely to succumb to peer pressure and do something he doesn't want to do than one who has a distant relationship with his parents.

If you do feel that peer pressure is influencing your child's view of his diabetes, try to work out why this should be. In Chapter 8, we talk about drinking, smoking and drugs and these are the obvious major problem areas. Perhaps your child's blood glucose levels are sky-high and you assume that he and his friends are continually eating sweets. What are you going to do about that? You certainly cannot stop your child's friends eating sweets or stop him seeing someone because they eat lots of sweets. Good diabetes education is far more likely to make him say 'no' when offered them. As 23-year-old Darren (who confesses that he's a 'teenager at heart') advises:

Eat a Mars bar and see how it affects your glucose levels. Is it really worth it? Then, learn how your insulin acts and how you can alter it to suit your needs.

As we explain in Chapter 6 on diet, sweet foods can be fitted into a healthy eating plan and can sometimes be used to help control diabetes (say, before exercise or to push up low blood glucose levels). Your teenager is far more likely to eat chocolate at the 'right' time and refuse it at the 'wrong' time if he understands how it can fit into his life, rather than seeing sweets as 'forbidden fruits'. In fact, these days, the majority of teenage girls are (rightly or wrongly) so conscious of staying slim that they tend to eat far fewer sweets and stodge than their parents did.

Whether or not peer pressure can have any other effect on your child's diabetes is debatable. It's highly unlikely that any of his friends would try to influence him not to take his insulin. If this were the case, he would soon realize that these were no kind of friends at all. So long as your child knows all the facts about diabetes (including the consequences of his actions), he will be able to sort out what's right and what's wrong for him. Without sounding callous, point out that diabetes is *his* condition and he must make the right decisions for the sake of his health.

If your teenager seems to be carrying on with his life as if he does not have diabetes, then he could well be in a state of denial about the whole thing. One mother who is understandably fraught with anxiety says:

> *Edward eats sweets and high-fat foods constantly, drinks ordinary cola, injects himself when he feels like it and never tests his blood glucose levels. In the year since he was diagnosed as having diabetes, he has turned into a monster – moody, rebellious about every little thing . . . Sometimes he's downright nasty. Am I the only mother of a child with diabetes who simply cannot accept that he has the condition?*

Edward's mother is not alone. Although so many of the teenagers who helped us with our survey had accepted their diabetes, learned to live with it and make it work for them, there are inevitably those who haven't yet managed to do this. But, with specialist help, they can come through this distressing period of denial and out the other side learning to come to terms with and accept their diabetes. In a situation such as Edward's mother describes, you should discuss the problem with your doctor or diabetes specialist nurse.

Sport and Exercise

One of the key factors in the balancing act for good blood glucose control is exercise, and in the case of the growing teenager, the more the better. Yet, some years ago, people with diabetes were completely discouraged from rigorous sport and exercise. Even in these enlightened times, there are still a number of misinformed souls who believe that this is still so and that someone with diabetes should not use up his energy. In short, he should be treated 'differently'. James, who is 18, reports:

> Some PE teachers do not allow students with diabetes to take part in sports because they are not educated enough about the condition. Luckily this has never happened to me and I decided to take a positive attitude and prove that diabetes does not stop you doing things . . . I now have many more activities than before I was diagnosed, including basketball, weight training, circuit training, trampolining and amateur motor racing.

Many teenagers have told us of the hair-raising activities they enjoyed while on BDA holidays (see Chapter 10), including canoeing, absailing, watersports, go-karting, paintballing and rock-climbing. An excellent introduction to sports that they may never have thought of trying even before they had diabetes gives youngsters the taste for more adventure. Jenny admits:

> Maybe I needed to show my friends I was no different from them. The funny thing is, now I am different . . . not because I have diabetes but because I'm crazy about wind-surfing (which I learned on a BDA holiday) and they've never had the chance to do it.

There's no doubt that exercise should be encouraged – it's fun, it's sociable and it keeps you fit. There are very few sports from which someone with diabetes should be discouraged, although a couple of teenagers in our survey complained that they had been banned from bungee jumping (probably to the great relief of their parents!) Until recently, scuba-diving, parachuting and motor racing were no-go areas, but we have heard that even these sports may be open now, subject to individual assessment. There are many sportsmen and women who have reached the top in all kinds of sports. There are also many marathon runners with diabetes who start and finish their races *and* are able to manage their blood glucose levels!

The fact is that lying in bed or in front of the TV is *not* good for blood glucose levels (or general fitness in anyone), as lounging around the house means that no energy is being used and the weight can pile on.

Cutting down insulin or eating some chocolate before exercise should help stop blood glucose levels from falling too low, while extended or indefinite periods of strenuous activity may need to be worked out by blood tests before and afterwards. Balancing blood glucose levels with insulin, food and exercise is very much a matter of trial and error, but the key to it, as we mentioned earlier, is blood testing. However much a teenager dislikes blood testing, it is wise for him to test before and after an activity as this gives an instant picture of whether insulin adjustment or carbohydrate intake is appropriate. Indeed, Gary Mabbutt – Spurs captain and former England player – tests before and after a football match, as well as at half time, topping up his glucose levels with Lucozade if necessary. It's important to find out what's going on in the body as blood glucose levels may not always be lowered *after* a bout of exercise.

When we exercise, the hormone adrenalin blocks the body's supply of insulin and, if there is not enough insulin circulating in the body in the first place, then there will be nothing to work on the glucose. If your teenager finds his blood glucose levels are high after exercise, this is a sign that he has not had enough insulin. Perhaps he has cut down his insulin dose in anticipation of the activity or is generally not having enough. Testing his blood will show that he needs more insulin in the preceeding dose and it will also tell him whether the exercise he took was as strenuous as he thought it would be. School PE lessons sometimes involve more standing around gossiping than real action, so he needs to be realistic about how much energy he *actually* uses as opposed to how much he *imagines* he uses. Hopefully, blood test-resisting teenagers will see the benefits of this if they are serious about their sport.

Different Types of Exercise

Running

Sprinting uses up a lot of energy in a short time and some rapidly absorbed carbohydrate (such as a glucose drink) will provide this energy. Afterwards, some more glucose and starchy carbohydrate will stop glucose levels falling too low.

Requirements for long-distance running are different as the exercise is taken over a far longer period. Instant energy (such as a glucose drink) is needed at the start, as is slowly absorbed (longer-lasting) starchy carbohydrate. If running cross-country or a marathon, intakes of instant energy will need to be repeated at intervals over the distance and, after the race, more glucose and plenty of starchy carbohydrate should be taken to stop falls in blood glucose levels occurring up to 24 hours later.

Running a marathon does not mean a person with diabetes has to appear to be any different to the other runners. If you've watched the London Marathon on TV, then you may have noticed participants pausing quite frequently for isotonic, or high energy drinks along the way, and many of them carry glucose tablets in the pockets of their shorts.

Swimming

Ideally your teenager should swim with a companion. That said, ensuring that enough carbohydrate has been eaten before the swim should eliminate any real risk of a hypo occurring while in the water.

If swimming in a public pool, your son or daughter should

always wear ID jewellery and, ideally, inform the lifeguard that he has diabetes (although the chances of a teenager doing this are minimal as most would regard it as 'making a fuss').

Watertight plastic containers worn around the neck are a good way of carrying glucose tablets – if they will wear one. However, if your teenager keeps glucose tablets handy near the side of the pool and leaves the water immediately he feels hypo warning signs, the risks of anything going wrong are slight. You must remember that a teenager will not *want* anything to go wrong and so long as he understands his requirements is unlikely to do anything to jeopardize his well-being or put himself in danger.

If swimming in the sea, your son or daughter should take all the precautions we've already described above, but also bear in mind the added hazards of large waves, dangerous currents and that swimming out too far from land could put him at great risk. He should certainly never risk swimming out to sea alone.

Weight Training

How much energy you expend training rather depends on the level of fitness you wish to achieve. Obviously, aerobic warm-ups burn energy faster and every individual varies in the amount they choose to do before and afterwards (cool-down). The only way of really knowing how much insulin should be reduced or carbohydrate taken is by testing before and after each session as building up the amount of exercise and weights may change requirements frequently.

Keep-fit Classes, Team Sports, Tennis and Others

All require some sugary carbohydrate beforehand and starchy carbohydrate afterwards, with something at half-time if the exercise is particularly strenuous.

Skiing

Wearing ID, warm clothes and packing plenty of food in a bumbag is the best advice here as the better your skiing, the further you are likely to end up from supplies left at the hotel or guest-house. Take insulin along, too, in case spontaneous eating forays are suggested (wrap the bottle or pen in insulating material to prevent the insulin freezing) and plenty of glucose tablets and mini chocolate bars to fuel all the energy required. Most people find that they have to cut their insulin by a third to half of their normal dose when skiing.

Going on Holiday

When a person is first diagnosed as having diabetes, they often cannot envisage travelling. Long journeys, time zone changes, jet-lag, foreign food, the heat, the cold, lack of medical facilities – sometimes the thought of it is all too daunting to contemplate. Charlie's mother, Liz, recalls:

> We had planned a trip to Florida when Charlie was taken ill and found to have diabetes. He was 11 at the time, the holiday was 6 weeks away and we were all in such a state that I phoned up the insurance company to ask about cancelling. I was advised to check with my doctor first as my broker assured me that several of his clients had diabetes and had been travelling happily for years. The doctor was most against us cancelling. 'There's no reason to call it off whatsoever,' he said. 'Apart from the fact that you'll find it easy to cope, think how Charlie would feel about missing the trip . . . and he'd feel guilty about messing up the family's plans.' We went and had a marvellous time.

There is no reason for diabetes to put a stop to holidays and travel. With some forward planning and anticipating potential problems, your son or daughter should be able to visit anywhere in the world, and, when he or she is old enough, without parents as travelling companions. Several of the older teenagers in our survey had been very adventurous, back-packing with friends around places such as India, Africa and the Far East. Parents, quite naturally, tended to be beside themselves with worry while their children were away, waiting anxiously for infrequent phone calls and letters that took an age to arrive, yet we heard of only one teenager who ended up in hospital. This was Peter, and he had his insulin supplies stolen in Thailand and developed a bad stomach infection before he could get hold of any more. Peter says:

I don't know why it should have suprised me, but the local doctor understood all about diabetes and sent me to hospital as an emergency. Even in this run-down hospital in the back of beyond, they had insulin.

Wherever he goes and whatever kind of holiday he chooses, your teenager should carry identification in both jewellery and card form. Wearing SOS/Talisman or Medic-Alert are advisable as opposed to dog-tags and so on as they are recognized all over the world. When abroad, it would certainly be wise to have an identification card written in the language of the country he is visiting. The BDA has a comprehensive pack with a wealth of information on this and other aspects of travel.

If your child needs to have vaccinations to visit certain countries, make sure he gets them done. Although vaccinations do not usually cause any particular problems in people with diabetes, he may find that they cause his glucose levels to rise and therefore needs some extra insulin to bring them back to normal. He should also have a letter from his doctor for customs saying that he has diabetes and that the syringes in his luggage do not mean he is a drug addict!

If travel sickness is a problem, your family GP will prescribe or recommend something to help. If he actually vomits, he should have sweetened fruit juice about every hour to replace carbohydrate foods he is unable to tolerate. Although he may vomit, ketosis will not develop – providing he does not stop his insulin – because once the travelling stops, so will the sickness (and blood tests will confirm what's going on). Extra short-acting insulin will stop blood glucose levels rising, and the diabetes specialist nurse will suggest an emergency dose plan.

A travelling teenager should make sure he eats regularly and always be prepared for delays by carrying plenty of glucose tablets and snacks, such as crisps, biscuits and sandwiches (chocolate is bound to melt), so there's no panic if mealtimes are delayed.

It's best to double-up on supplies when travelling – insulin, syringes, testing strips and lancets. If your teenager uses a pen, he should take a spare one and even some disposable syringes in case the pen(s) get lost or broken. He can use syringes to draw up insulin from the cartridges that usually go in the pen, but should *not* put air into the cartridge before drawing up or else the rubber bung at the end will fly off. Even if he uses pre-mixed insulin, he should still take a bottle of short-acting insulin in case of illness. One complete set of equipment should be carried in his hand-luggage, the other with a travelling companion who can be trusted not to lose it. He should not allow anyone else to take it away, even for safekeeping, and the equipment should always be within easy reach – that includes hypostoppers, snacks and so on. If, however, he is travelling alone, he should put duplicate equipment in a jacket pocket or traveller's belt.

Note that insulin should never be put in the hold of an aircraft as it will freeze (also, it is not unknown for luggage to end up in a totally different location to the one you're going to!) It will remain stable out of the fridge for a month as long as it is not exposed to direct sunlight or heat. A Thermos flask or small insulated bag can also be used if the weather is warm. Ice in the thermos may make insulin freeze. Even in hot countries it can be kept wrapped in cool flannels at the back of a drawer or wardrobe.

If he uses a glucose-testing meter which has test-strips that cannot also be colour-matched to a chart by eye, then he should allow for the fact that his meter may break or become lost and ask his doctor for a brand of strips that can be read by eye alone (or buy a meter using strips that can be read both electronically *and* by eye). Some meters do not work above or below certain temperatures, so check the manufacturers' instructions.

Most countries follow the same principles for diabetes care as in the UK. However, if your teenager is not travelling with you, he should check that his insurance covers the fact that he has diabetes (most do allow for this). If travelling in Europe, he should complete form E111 from the DHSS. Some countries do not use U100 insulin (as we do), they use U40, which can only be drawn up in

U40 syringes. Nevertheless, a comparable insulin to the one your teenager uses should be available if the worst happens and his supplies are lost or stolen. The BDA can provide further information on insulin and diabetes care in different countries.

Here is a checklist of everything your teenager will need for travelling, either in this country or abroad (as mentioned earlier, it is sensible to duplicate all the equipment):

- insulin
- syringes
- pen
- testing strips (and meter if used), pricking device and lancets
- log book for blood/urine test results
- ketone testing strips
- glucagon and/or Hypostop
- ID jewellery and card
- glucose tablets, snacks, flask or coolbox/bag
- form E111 from main post offices if travelling inside the EU
- a letter from the doctor stating that he has diabetes and identification in the language of the country he is visiting.

It's true that airlines will provide a special diabetic meal if ordered in advance, but these, frankly, are best avoided as they contain little or no carbohydrate. It's best to stick to the normal meal provided and supplement it with snacks and fruit juice if it proves (as they often do), inedible.

A teenager should also be aware that hot weather can affect blood glucose control, causing insulin to be absorbed more quickly, which may lead to hypos. He may find that he needs to reduce his dose of insulin or have injections nearer his meal. As usual, blood testing will give the answers and, even if your child is anti blood testing, he will hopefully appreciate that while he is away from home he should be ultra-responsible and gauge how he is reacting to the differences in weather, activities and food.

Anna tells us:

You get used to coping in really difficult circumstances once you've done a bit of travelling without the nannying of your parents. It becomes a real challenge, and I can tell you that being stuck in the Australian outback is a real survival special! But, for me, overcoming difficulties without a major fuss being made is one of the most challenging and rewarding things about having diabetes. Sure you're different . . . but you're also resourceful, brave and never short of a story to tell!

Chapter 6

DIET: HEALTHY FOODS, JUNK FOODS AND EATING DISORDERS

If your teenager has recently been diagnosed as having diabetes, you may be confused as to what she should or should not be eating. The hospital dietitian will have explained that your child can stick to a normal, healthy diet – one that is high in fibre, low in fat, low in sugar and has lots of complex carbohydrates. Yet, if you have never known anyone with diabetes before now, you may feel uneasy about this. Many of the teenagers and parents in our survey commented on well-meaning souls who appeared to think that anything containing sugar was now off the menu:

I thought people with diabetes collapsed if they ate sugar.

I went round to my friend's house for tea and her mum rushed around hiding the biscuits. We all ate cheese sandwiches and I started to feel hypo. I asked for a chocolate biscuit and she said I should call the doctor.

Before everything had been explained to me properly, I told Suzy that she would never be able to eat chocolate again.

I ordered some ice-cream in a restaurant and my grandmother told the waiter to cancel it, saying, 'She's diabetic you see . . .'

It's quite understandable that generations of people who grew up before and during the 1960s are baffled as it's only in the last 20 years or so that the thinking as to what a person with diabetes should eat has changed completely. Before the discovery of insulin, someone who suffered from diabetes would be virtually starved to give them any chance of survival. Their life may have been prolonged for a short while in this way, but they succumbed to malnutrition eventually.

Even with the advent of insulin replacement, starchy and sugary carbohydrates were severely restricted, with the recommended diet consisting mainly of fat and protein – and plenty of it – to satisfy the voracious appetite. The high rate of heart and kidney problems in people with diabetes that resulted showed that something was badly wrong and it became clear that carbohydrate could not be cited as the culprit simply because so little was being consumed by those with diabetes.

Intensive research showed that a diet including a high proportion of starchy carbohydrate and fibre reduced levels of fat in the blood, which were being linked to heart disease. When home blood glucose monitoring became available, it was seen on a day-to-day basis that control of diabetes could be considerably improved and the 'new' food plan recommended to the population as a whole took the place of what had previously been known as the 'diabetic diet'.

Where to Begin

If your teenager has previously been used to a lot of sugary food and drink, then these should certainly be cut down and replaced with low-sugar substitutes or products containing artificial sweeteners. Apart from the important aspect of her blood glucose control, this is far better for the youngster's teeth and general health. However, chocolate or ice-cream would be perfectly acceptable at certain times, such as after a high-fibre meal, before exercise or if blood glucose is low.

Special 'diabetic' foods, such as chocolates, cakes, biscuits, jams and so on are not in any way necessary – or worth including – in your child's diet. Sugar is replaced by what are known as bulk sweeteners that are not low in calories ('bulk' because they are used in similar quantities to sugar, as opposed to low-calorie sweeteners which are used in very small amounts), and the products often contain a high proportion of fat to make them palatable. These items are therefore as high – or higher – in calories as most ordinary products and can still affect the blood glucose because of the bulk sweeteners. Incidentally, consuming large amounts of these products can cause a nasty bout of the runs! In these days of health-conscious eating, the market is awash with low-sugar and low-fat foods that people with diabetes can enjoy and so there is no need at all for these calorific and expensive 'diabetic' products. Indeed, the BDA stopped advertising them in its magazine some time ago.

A clear idea of how foods are broken down in the body may help your teenager to understand what the hospital dietitian is really talking about when he or she advocates a 'sensible eating plan'. Some teenagers admitted that they only half understood what was being said on their first visit to the dietitian. Perhaps they found the whole idea of rethinking their diet so horrific they rejected certain information out of hand without even taking it in.

Until she really bothered to find out exactly which foods contained fibre and why they were so important, Sally rejected her dietitian's advice:

She mentioned 'pulses' and 'lentils' and that put me off straightaway! Perhaps I wasn't paying attention or simply didn't want to know, but I took it that the only foods that were any good for me were those cranky things that vegetarians go on about, so I carried on eating my fry-ups and greasy chips. It was only when we had a lesson in nutrition at school and I had to write an essay on which foods contained fibre and how they benefit digestion that I realized I could change my diet to low-fat, high-fibre without becoming some kind of beancurd bore.

The Way Foods Work

In order to make the body work correctly, it is necessary to choose foods from three main groups:

- carbohydrates
- fats
- protein.

Carbohydrates provide energy. Fats also provide energy and are stored as energy reserves, as well as being an important source of vitamins. Protein enables the cells and tissues in the body to grow and repair themselves.

Some of the foods we eat fall into just one of these groups, such as bread, which is mainly carbohydrate, but, in many foods, the groups overlap. A good example of this is milk, which contains carbohydrate, fat *and* protein. It is the proportions of these different foods in our diet that is important and, as a guide, about half the energy in our diets should come from carbohydrate foods, no more than a third from fat and a little from protein.

Carbohydrates Explained

Carbohydrates directly affect the treatment and control of diabetes and therefore have the most significant place in your teenager's diet. There are two types of carbohydrate:

- sugary
- starchy.

Sugary carbohydrates cause a sharp rise in glucose levels, due to the rapid way they are digested by the body, and, apart from using them to treat hypos or as an energy booster before exercise, they have no nutritional virtues.

It is for this reason that sugary foods should not be a regular part of your teenager's diet, but they can, by all means, be included as treats. Quite often, people who develop diabetes manage to wean themselves off sugary foods and then cannot stand the taste of them at all and instead of chocolate being a treat, it turns into something they only eat when they have to.

Starchy carbohydrates, however, are digested more slowly by the body, causing a much smaller rise in the blood glucose level. Including regular portions of these foods through the day (that is, some at each meal), means that the blood glucose level stays up but doesn't go too high – which is exactly what you're aiming for. Bread, potatoes, pasta, rice and breakfast cereals are all starchy foods.

Foods that are High in Fibre

There has been a lot of publicity about the benefits of including high-fibre foods in the diet for some years now and you may already include many foods containing fibre in your family's meals as a matter of course. Baked potatoes, wholemeal bread, fruit, vegetables and good old baked beans, are the norm in many households. If this is the case, your teenager will be used to eating a number of high-fibre foods.

Fibre slows down the rate at which sugar is absorbed into the blood and so helps to keep the blood glucose levels under control. There are lots of simple changes that can be made so that more high-fibre foods are included on a regular basis. White bread, chips and cereals that are low in fibre can be easily substituted for alternatives that are higher in fibre. Look out for wholemeal or wholewheat on the labels in products such as breads and cereals. Note that brown, wheatgerm and wheatmeal are *not* high-fibre products.

If your child hates the thought of eating wholemeal bread, there are white breads available that contain more fibre, such as the multigrain varieties. Try wholegrain rice rather than polished rice and replace white pasta with the wholemeal variety. As for cereals, Shredded Wheat, Weetabix, Fruit and Fibre and Ready-Brek are all popular with youngsters and are much higher in fibre than Rice Crispies or Corn Flakes. Use an artificial sweetener for those who like their cereals to be sweet-tasting. Cereals can also be sweetened with raw or dried fruit, such as sultanas, apricots or sliced banana.

Vegetables and pulses are excellent sources of fibre, and pulses include kidney beans, butter beans, lentils, chickpeas and, of course, the haricot beans that are smothered in tomato sauce and known as baked beans! Beans used to be a bit of a hassle years ago, due to the overnight soaking or pre-cooking that they required, but now there is a huge variety of ready-to-use beans in tins at the supermarkets. It's easy to throw the contents of a tin into a Bolognese sauce, chilli or casserole or to use them in a salad.

Fruits are an invaluable source of fibre. Fruits contain their own sugars (fructose), but, in most cases, the sugar content is small and tied up with fibre, so it is more slowly absorbed into the bloodstream than table sugar (sucrose) would be. Encourage your teenager to eat plenty of fruit, but suggest that they eat it throughout the day rather than eat lots in one go, as this can put the sugars up.

Pure fruit juices can be a problem as the juice is highly concentrated. They do not contain the fibre that fresh fruit has so they are absorbed into the bloodstream quite quickly. Teenagers often like to drink fruit juice in large quantities and may find it hard to accept that diabetes now restricts them in this. You could point out that they would be better off drinking their favourite juice as an accompaniment to a meal rather than on its own or dilute it with fizzy water. If you make sure you keep regular supplies in the house of diet squash and diet versions of their favourite fizzy drinks, then, hopefully, there shouldn't be too much complaining. Incidentally, because of the high amount of fructose in concentrated fruit juices, they are ideal if your son or daughter feels a hypo coming on.

Fats and Fatty Foods

Everyone needs *some* fat in their diet and it would be almost impossible to cut it out completely, but it is important to cut down on the overall amount of fat that we eat. This is especially important for people with diabetes for two reasons. The first is that cutting down on fat helps to avoid becoming overweight, which can make diabetes more difficult to control (fat contains twice as many calories per ounce as carbohydrate and protein), and the second is that it can reduce the risk of developing heart disease and circulation problems.

Heart disease is quite hard for most teenagers to relate to as it is usually something that happens to 'old' people, so they don't understand why it should worry them now. On the one hand they *shouldn't* worry about it, but, on the other, good habits developed now will usually carry on into adulthood and protect them from this possibility.

The newly diagnosed person with diabetes has a lot to cope with, trying to get to grips with all the information about sugars and starches and regular meals, so take it easy with the subject of cutting down on fat. Don't expect your teenager to go from an average chips and crisps teenager to a pulse-eating, fruit fan overnight – it takes time to change ingrained eating habits.

Here are some simple tips for ways in which you can cut down your intake of fat:

- avoid frying or roasting food or having fried foods, such as chips
- use less or no spread on bread
- eat less cheese and processed meats, such as sausages, pork pies, corned beef.
- use a semi-skimmed or skimmed milk
- have fewer fatty snacks and take-away meals (often particularly relevant for teenagers).

Saturated v. Unsaturated Fat

It's easy to become confused by the saturated fat/cholesterol/olive oil arguments as there appears to be so much conflicting information around – and this is not helped by food manufacturers, whose job it is to sell products rather than to educate.

In a nutshell, a high fat intake has been shown to increase the risk of heart disease (and becoming overweight, which is a risk factor in its own right) and the more 'harmful' type of fat is the saturated kind, which is generally animal fat, such as that found in butter or lard. Cutting down on the total fat consumed will decrease this risk, so this is the most important thing to do. However, it is also important to note that the fat you *do* eat should be unsaturated fat, which is found in sunflower margarine and olive oil, for example.

Here is a shopping guide:

- avoid butter, lard and dairy spreads, which are very high in saturated fats
- unsaturated fats can be polyunsaturated or monosaturated and these are the names to look out for on spreads and oils in phrases such as 'high in polyunsaturates'
- only spreads that specify that they are 'low fat' actually *are* low in fat (other margarines have the same fat content as butter), so buying low-fat spreads is a better idea
- blended vegetable oils often contain a lot of saturated fat, so buy an oil of a specific variety, such as sunflower, olive, corn
- all vegetable oils are low in cholesterol so do not get confused by this term on unsaturated oils and spreads.

Really though, in the end, it is the amount you use that is important, rather than the type you buy!

Protein Foods

Protein is essential for growth, which means all teenagers should have sufficient protein in their diets as they are still growing. However, it is true that most people eat more protein than they actually need, so there is usually no need to encourage a large intake of protein foods.

Protein is contained in meat and fish, dairy products, such as eggs, cheese and milk, and in alternatives like beans, lentils, Quorn and tofu. Providing your son or daughter is eating a portion of these foods two or three times a day, they should be getting sufficient protein. Another reason for not eating too much protein is that the foods in this group often also contain a fair bit of fat – as is the case for cheese or fatty meats (and it is mainly *saturated* fat) – so keeping the intake of protein down helps keep the consumption of fats down as well.

To Sum Up

Meals should be regular and based on starchy foods, as these provide energy as well as keeping the blood glucose steady. Starchy foods should be high in fibre where possible. The meat portion should be fairly small and it should be lean, and the vegetable and fruit portions should be fairly big.

What About Junk Foods?

'It's all very well having lots of healthy food in the house . . . but my son eats nothing but junk when he goes out!', says Lesley, mother of 15-year-old Tony.

As many parents of teenagers know, once their offspring are out and about, away from the routine of home-cooking, all sorts of so-called unwholesome eating rituals take place. Junk foods, fast foods, rubbish foods – however you refer to them – these are health-conscious parents' nightmare. Yet, is fast food really *all* bad?

Actually, it's not as bad as you may think, and if your teenager is able to appreciate which of her favourite fast foods are better than others and why, she can be more selective about her choices. Let's look at the nutritional value of some of the commonest fast foods.

Chinese

Chinese meals can be high in fat when dishes such as pork balls, spring rolls and so on are chosen. But, most stir-fried dishes are an OK bet, providing they are served with rice (boiled rather than egg fried, preferably) or noodles as the carbohydrate component.

Chips or French Fries

A staple in the diets of many teenagers, all chips and fries are high in fat, so no particular ones are better than others. However, it's worth bearing the following points in mind. Chippy-style chips are thick cut so absorb less oil than thin fries (as the ratio of outer surface to the potato inside is less), but are usually sold in large portions. As most people can eat more potato cooked as chips than if they were, say, boiled or baked, eating chips may result in raised blood glocose because an unusually high amount of carbohydrate has been consumed.

Thin fries, on the other hand (like those produced in burger chains), absorb more fat, but the portions tend to be smaller and therefore a little more controlled.

Donar Kebabs

The pitta bread provides the carbohydrate, but the meat can sometimes be on the greasy side. Choosing to have lots of salad and a little less meat (just ask) can improve things.

Fried Chicken or Fish

This kind of fast food is the one highest in fat. Fried chicken and fish are more fat-laden than hamburgers as they are deep-fried in batter. They need to be served with chips to provide a decent amount of carbohydrate, and so they are a very high-fat meal.

Hamburgers

Burgers are usually cooked on a griddle, so large amounts of fat do not need to be used for cooking. Choosing a plain burger with lots of salad rather than cheese or mayonnaise is the healthiest option and the bun will provide carbohydrate. Up-market burger restaurants often offer jacket potatoes or potato skins (these *are* fried, but the inclusion of the skins means they are higher in fibre than chips) which are a good alternative to French fries.

Hot Dogs

Frankfurters, like all sausages, are high in fat. The roll provides some carbohydrate, so they are OK as a quick snack, but probably not sufficient as a meal on their own.

Indian

This is not fast food as such, but is often a convenient late-evening option. The majority of Indian food served in restaurants is high in fat, even the vegetable dishes. Better choices are those such as tandoori and tikka dishes as they are not coated in a high-fat sauce or deep-fried. Also, drier dishes, such as biryanis, are a better bet than the creamier curries (kormas and massalas). Vegetarian dishes, although oily, often use lentils or chickpeas and therefore have some fibre in them. As accompaniments, plain rice – as opposed to pilau or fried – and naan bread provide good forms of carbohydrate.

Jacket Potatoes

These really are a good choice (so long as they are not smothered in butter and/or cheese). There are quite a few chains specializing in jacket potatoes, and visiting these can only be encouraged!

Pasta

Many restaurant chains have opened up over the last few years that serve cheap and cheerful pasta dishes, and these are a perfect choice for your teenager.

Cheese and cream-laden sauces should be avoided, but most young people love spaghetti Bolognese, lasagne, ravioli and so on, and many of the tomato-based sauces are very tempting.

Pizza

Made in the proper Italian way – thin, with a small amount of cheese – these can be very nutritious. It is the American-style, deep-pan pizza with lots of cheese and fatty meat toppings (salami, pepperoni) that are high in fat. Most teenagers tend to visit the American-style pizza chains, so encourage them to opt for thin bases with lots of *vegetable* toppings – and why not have a side salad rather then garlic bread? With some thought, this can be a reasonably healthy meal.

Snacking

Even if they don't happen to have a sweet tooth, teenagers are notorious 'grazers' of savoury snacks and these may well have a high fat content. Or, if they do have a sweet tooth, it is difficult for them to know what to snack on that is low in sugar. If you shop for healthier types of snacks so that your teenager gets the taste for them, then she may be more inclined to buy low-fat, low-sugar snacks when she's out. Even if she doesn't, though, her intake of high-fat snacks will be reduced considerably by eating in a more healthy way at home. Here is a look at the pros and cons of some of the commonest snacks teenagers choose.

Biscuits

One of the most common snacks for teenagers. Regular snacks of chocolate and cream-filled varieties should be avoided, but fairly plain biscuits are fine. Biscuits do contain some sugar and fat though, so the crunchy bread-type snacks mentioned below are good alternatives.

Cakes and Buns

Eating sweet cakes, doughnuts, pastries, croissants and so on on a regular basis should be avoided. However, there are lots of lower sugar alternatives available that are likely to be enjoyed just as much. Examples are bagels, bran muffins, crumpets, wholemeal fruit buns, teacakes and savoury scones.

Cereal Bars

They have a fair bit of sugar in them but a fair bit of fibre, too, so are a good choice.

Cereal and Toast

Don't forget these staple foods as snacks. Readily available at home, if they are high-fibre varieties then so much the better, and they are particularly good as a long-lasting bedtime snack.

Chocolate

Most people love chocolate and, because of this, there is no need to deny a little chocolate now and again. It is particularly good to use as a before-exercise boost, and the mini-size bars now available are a nice size to use.

There are some low-calorie chocolate bars around that are really just a smaller or puffed rice-filled version of the standard type of chocolate bars we are used to. So, while these might be an excellent idea to satisfy a craving now and again – don't be fooled by the marketing!

Crisps and Similar Packet Snacks

These contain no sugar but are high in fat. Reduced-fat varieties are now available, and are therefore a better choice than other varieties on a regular basis.

Crunchy Bread-style Snacks

Low-fat pretzels, crackers, Italian breadsticks and rice cakes are all very good 'grazing' foods.

Mousses and Ice-cream

Check the labelling carefully here. Diet or 'lite' varieties are low in fat *and* sugar (often containing artificial sweetener) whereas low- or no-fat products often contain lots of sugar to boost the taste.

Nuts

Nuts do not contain carbohydrates but they are high in fat. They are therefore no good as a snack designed to top up sugars in between meals so eating handfuls of peanuts ad lib (and aren't they moreish?) is not a good idea because of the fat. However, mixing nuts with some dried fruit can make a useful in-between snack, and a little peanut butter spread on wholemeal toast is a less fattening way to satisfy that craving for nuts.

Popcorn

A good nibbling snack, as plain popcorn is fairly low in carbohydrate. It's best to make your own and then you can use less butter for 'popping'. An even better method is using the microwave variety, which means no fat is used at all. Sweeten with artificial sweetener if required.

Yoghurts and Fromage Frais

Diet varieties of these are excellent snacks and desserts as they are low in fat and sugar. Keep the fridge well stocked with them! Remember, though, varieties that only say they are low in fat are not low in sugar. So, if in doubt, check the label.

Snacking Tip

The best idea with snacks is to vary them so that it doesn't matter if one snack is a little higher in sugar or another is higher in fat. Variety also prevents boredom, too, particularly in those who need to snack several times a day.

There's no point in getting uptight because your teenager has not lost her sweet tooth or refuses to give up chocolate. Arguments are only going to lead to secret sweet eating and an unwillingness to divulge any information about what she buys when she's out. As Emma tells us:

My mum nearly drove me crazy telling me what I shouldn't be eating and tut-tutting if she found me at the biscuit tin. I became so fed up with this one Christmas that I collected a drawerful of chocolate selection boxes and spent an evening eating my way through them. I ended up being very sick on Christmas day and having a dreadful row about how much I resented my diabetes and most of all, my mum for being such a pain in the neck.

If this is happening in your home, all we can advise is that you should stop, take several paces back from the situation and try to understand that you are almost certainly doing more harm than good. Take a low-key approach, buying acceptable options for eating at home. In the end, your teenager has to take responsibility for what she eats and must make her own choices. You can remind her that sweet foods are better absorbed after a high-fibre meal and her favourites can be eaten before exercise or when her blood glucose levels are low. Overall, it is healthy eating that you are aiming for, which generally means that nothing sweet or fatty is banned, just better eaten less often!

Eating Disorders

You will no doubt have heard of the eating disorders anorexia nervosa and bulimia as they seem to have had much coverage in the media over the last few years. It is an unfortunate fact that some people with diabetes (notably teenage girls, although it seems to be increasingly common in boys these days) are so used to watching the carbohydrate and fat content of the food they eat, that dieting can turn into an obsession.

Weight control can be especially difficult for a girl with diabetes who often eats more than she may have wanted in order to avoid her blood glucose levels falling too low. If you notice a weight problem looming on the horizon, it may be best to suggest visiting the hospital dietitian and diabetes nurse who will be able to advise on cutting down food and insulin successfully and safely. This should pre-empt the teenager taking matters into her own hands and possibly going too far. Sometimes, however, you just can't see a problem coming, as Beth's mother recalls:

Beth's problem started around four years ago, when she was 16. She had been diagnosed as having diabetes at eight but had always enjoyed her food, eating a high-fibre, low-fat diet quite happily. She had no weight problem – she was a size ten – but the trouble started when she was put on the Pill as she suffered from bad premenstrual syndrome. The doctor told her that she would probably put on weight as a result of the Pill and there was no way Beth was going to let this happen. Low fat became no fat. She cut her insulin to a quarter of her usual dose and ate virtually nothing. She knew she had to keep up her carbohydrate intake to stop herself becoming hypo so a 'meal' consisted of two slices of dried bread. I knew something was wrong when I realized how much she'd reduced her insulin and exactly what food she existed on. She became fanatical about her blood sugars; if she had a blood test of 12, she wouldn't eat at all.

Once the doctor realized that Beth had an eating disorder, he admitted her to hospital, but all they did was try and force her to eat high-fat foods and drink full-cream milk which we hadn't had in the house for years. Of course, this went against what she knew she was supposed to eat for her diabetes control and she became aggressive, angry . . . the whole thing was a nightmare. What Beth really needed was counselling, someone to talk through her problems, be understanding and help her.

I've spoken to quite a few other parents in our area's BDA support group. A number of people have teenagers with eating disorders and have also found a complete lack of back-up as far as emotional or psychological symptoms go. Beth is better about her eating habits now, but I can't help feeling that the support of a good psychologist

– who didn't just try and force her to eat – would have been in-valuable and that makes me very angry.

Beth's mother's story is a serious cause for concern as eating disorders are now better understood and therefore treated as serious emotional problems. Below are outlines of the main eating disorders to be aware of.

Anorexia Nervosa

When a child is anorexic, avoiding food becomes an obsession. Often, excessive exercise is taken to burn extra calories and laxatives may be used to boost weight loss. Losing weight makes the teenager feel good. Even when she is, in reality, gaunt and ultra-thin, she only sees herself as fat – a distorted self-image. She is usually intensely interested in food and most knowledgeable about nutritional values of everything, yet the idea of actually eating fills her with disgust.

In mild cases, anorexia causes loss of muscle strength, nutritional deficiencies and hormonal imbalances (periods usually stop because of this). There will be increased susceptibility to infection.

The warning signs are:

- actual fear of putting on weight and becoming fat
- talking incessantly about weight, calories and so on
- extreme weight loss (being 25 per cent below the weight that is normal for their height and age)
- drastic reduction of insulin and an avoidance of any explanation as to why it has been reduced
- distorted body image – claiming to feel fat even when emaciated
- total denial that there is a problem
- frequent hypos may point to little food being eaten
- an avid interest in calorific values of foods, even making elaborate meals for others but not eating them themselves, usually giving the excuse that they have already eaten.

Bulimia

Out of the two main types of eating disorder, bulimia has (until recently) been the lesser known. Now we're told that Princess Diana suffers from bulimia and suddenly it appears to have become better understood and mentioned far more frequently in the media.

Unlike people with anorexia, those with bulimia tend to stay within a normal weight range and some are even overweight, so the condition is far harder to detect. Also, whereas the anorexic's strict regime of non-eating makes her feel in control, the pattern of the bulimic's behaviour makes her feel very much the opposite.

The classic pattern of bulimia is uncontrollable bingeing in a short space of time, with thousands of calories consumed in an hour, followed by self-induced vomiting to eliminate the unwanted calories. Some people with bulimia may binge for a fortnight, then starve for weeks afterwards. Bulimics are tormented by their eating habits and, although they might appear outward-going and stable, their secretive side harbours depression, feelings of worthlessness and self-disgust.

Bulimia appears to be found more often than anorexia in people with diabetes, and perhaps it is caused psychologically by there being a denial of their condition in that they will binge on unsuitable foods. This will often be followed by feeling guilty for eating these particular foods and the inevitable vomiting.

The warning signs of bulimia are:

- stores of food hidden in the teenager's bedroom
- suspicion that vomiting has been self-induced, evidence of use of laxatives, periodic dieting or fasting
- abnormal swings in blood glucose levels
- generally secretive and erratic behaviour.

Midmed Syndrome

Midmed refers to 'the manipulation of insulin dose as the manifestation of an eating disorder'. It could also be described as diabetic bulimia as midmed syndrome is a specific but not uncommon problem that can only affect people with diabetes.

In this case, the teenager does not need to make herself vomit as she knows that constantly high blood glucose can cause weight loss and she is able to binge – usually on sweet foods – so her insulin dose cannot cover her food intake. Thus, she is hyperglycaemic and may show ketones in her urine when she wants to lose weight.

Sophie explains:

I spent a long time going through cycles of bingeing to satisfy my craving for sweet foods. I didn't want to make myself vomit or take laxatives and I didn't have to. I could manipulate my insulin to keep myself alive and out of a coma . . . Admittedly, I felt unwell – always thirsty and passing urine . . . but I could lose up to 10 pounds in a couple of weeks, then go back to more normal blood sugars for a while. I became very ill in the end and had to be hospitalized.

After counselling, I realized that I couldn't go on this way and the psychologist and dietitian helped me with a proper diet plan, which I'm sticking to. I hope I've put the bingeing behind me for good.

The warning signs of this condition are:

- symptoms of high blood glucose levels with sudden weight loss
- long-term blood test results (HbA1C) being high and not matching those recorded at home
- hidden stores of food, secretive and erratic behaviour
- general ill-health, perhaps with frequent infections or thrush.

What to Do

Fortunately, there are many doctors and nurses specializing in diabetes who realize that anorexia and bulimia can be a major problem among teenagers and who take immediate action by referring them to a psychologist (or psychiatrist) for the right help. If you suspect that your child is reducing her insulin and food beyond the limits of normal dieting or find evidence that she is bingeing, vomiting or using laxatives, then she needs immediate attention from experts in this field.

Please don't be alarmed by the above outlines of eating disorders and feel that, because diabetes is such a food-orientated condition, it is inevitable that your teenage daughter (or son) will succumb. The statistics are that 7 per cent more people with diabetes than those who do not have diabetes have some kind of eating disorder, yet, as with all self-inflicted problems in life, there are certain people who are susceptible and there are no hard and fast rules as to why this should happen to any particular in-dividual, whether they have diabetes or not. All we are trying to say is, be aware.

Chapter 7

PROBLEMS AND HASSLES

However well your teenager copes with diabetes, there are bound to be times when, as 17-year-old Andrew put it, 'It's a complete pain in the backside'. Although injections, blood tests and eating regularly become an inconvenience of life, perhaps the real acid test is when things go wrong socially and prejudice is encountered as then the youngster is forced to face certain problems head-on and learn how to deal with them without giving up his goals and wallowing in self-pity.

The majority of people do not see that there is any stigma attached to diabetes – most of the old-fashioned fear and prejudice went out with the boiling of glass syringes. However, we wouldn't be talking real life if we maintained that there is no bigotry or intolerance around. As with anything different, narrow-minded and/or ignorant people will exist. In this chapter, therefore, we look at some examples of the hassles encountered by the teenagers in our survey, which are, hopefully, balanced by positive solutions to certain problems.

Relationships

Amanda, aged 15, told us:

I once got friendly with a guy called Chris and we were going great until he brought me a Mars bar. Well, I'd just eaten a big meal so I couldn't have it. I told him I had diabetes and the look on his face . . . I'll never forget it! The bottom dropped out of my world. I think he expected me to turn green and explode or something so I explained the basics to him. I could tell he just wasn't going to be comfortable when we were together so I forgot about him.

It's happened a couple of times and you soon learn that, however much you think you like someone, if they can't handle the situation, then they're not worth bothering about. I was really upset when it happened with Chris, but I've learned that a true friend is someone who is interested in every aspect about you and I'm very secure with those friendships that I have.

Mark has had similar experiences:

Most of my friends are aware that I have diabetes and don't treat me any differently. But I'm reluctant to tell people who don't know me very well as I've found in the past that they dismissed me as being trouble before they could understand that having diabetes wouldn't restrict me from doing anything that they wanted to do.

Perhaps the solution is to take time to show the doubters how diabetes can fit in with a normal life. Charlotte, mother of Harry (now aged 13) did just that:

When Harry was diagnosed, I found that social invitations dried up. His friend's parents seemed scared stiff to have him in the house, let alone have him stay the night! This was both frustrating and depressing, so, in the end, I organized a sleepover party. That did the trick as the other boys reported back to their parents that Harry was eating, running around and behaving in exactly the same wild way as his mates. Nothing dreadful happened in the night . . . he showed them how it took precisely half a minute to do his injection, didn't take him an hour to recover and he ate the same foods as everyone else without collapsing in a heap. In other words, the parents were informed that he was quite normal. Since then, the invitations haven't stopped.

Seventeen-year-old Susie says:

In my experience, most people are fascinated by diabetes and admire you for having to do the injections. I also think that people feel they know you better if they are aware of your diabetes. If a boyfriend or girlfriend dumps you because of it, then they are definitely not worth bothering about.

Sam, 15, agrees:

Your diabetes is only the tip of the iceberg. If someone can't be doing with that, just think how uncaring and selfish they would be about everything else in a relationship. Diabetes can provide a lucky escape before you become too involved with a rat.

As you will read in Chapter 10, the BDA provides many opportunities for young people with diabetes to meet in all kinds of situations, ranging from weekend discussion groups to skiing trips, and these occasions are extremely popular. However, there are those who prefer not to mix with such a group. Fourteen-year-old Katy admits:

I don't like being labelled as a 'minority'. It's not really the diabetes . . . I didn't like being a Brownie and I prefer people don't know I'm Jewish, either.

Yet, the general feeling is that meeting other youngsters in the same boat can promote self-confidence, especially in the early days after diagnosis. Naomi told us that one of her 12-year-old daughter's closest friendships was formed on the basis of both children having diabetes:

When Suzy was diagnosed five years ago, she was introduced to Harry (who is a year older) by a mutual friend. It turned out his family lived round the corner, yet we'd never met. At first, their friendship was wary – perhaps they felt they were being pushed together. But, after a while, it took off and they became best buddies. They hardly discuss their diabetes at all but, as both will maintain, 'we understand each other'.

Sadly, Harry's family has moved to another part of the country now, but we still see them regularly and the bond will always be there. Suzy has met other children with diabetes through our local support group, but has never been interested in pursuing these friendships. The rest of her friends do not have diabetes and to them she is absolutely normal, but, I'm sure, Harry will always be special to her.

School Problems

A very small number of parents and teenagers have encountered problems in the form of verbal bullying at school, usually because the child needs to eat extra snacks when others are not allowed them. Rebecca – now 17 – recalls:

When I first started secondary school, one particular girl gave me a hard time about the snacks I had to eat before games. She told me I was greedy and that I was using my diabetes to get attention from everyone. She also told me I was fat, which was stupid because I was much slimmer than her. After a while, the comments really got to me and I told my mum, who went to see the teacher. She was quite shocked and took the opportunity of explaining diabetes to the class during a biology lesson, directing most of the information at this girl. She asked her if she would like to see what it's like to have a needle stuck in her body four times a day. She declined . . . there was no problem after that.

One of Debbie's teachers amazed her by saying, 'Diabetes doesn't seem to have affected your intelligence'.

Such incidences are pretty few and far between, usually arising out of ignorance because the child with diabetes had not made their condition known or because teachers had not fully explained the reasons for 'snacking' to the class. Clear explanations to the guilty parties inevitably result in remorse and an end to the problem. In one or two cases, the offending party has been moved to a different class or parents were called in. In all cases, careful handling by teachers puts a stop to any distress.

Tony's teacher was quick off the mark when a rumour began circulating among the 11-year-olds that both diabetes and asthma were contagious:

Myself and three other boys were told by some others that we couldn't hang around with them in case they caught something from us. Our form tutor couldn't believe it! He dealt with the situation very well and gave a talk to the class, pointing out in no uncertain terms that diabetes and asthma were not catching but ignorance was! He didn't even mention our names, but afterwards everyone apologized to us and we've never had any more trouble.

Fear of being teased or rejected through ignorance can be devastating. Indeed, it prevented Tom (now 15) from attending school altogether when he was diagnosed two years ago. His mother, Sue (who was then found to have insulin-dependent diabetes herself), told us:

He can't face having any attention re. the diabetes from his peers and has missed nearly 18 months of school. He is now very withdrawn and isolated but is soon to start a programme of being integrated back into school.

Sadly, we are aware of the poor attitude some teachers have towards their pupils who have diabetes. One headteacher intimated that Simon should attend a special school where he would have the attention he required. Even though Simon's diabetes nurse talked to her and explained that this was, of course, totally unnecessary, she maintained her ignorant attitude. If your teenager has had to put up with such ridiculous ignorance and unhelpfulness, then you should perhaps consider sorting out the problem by changing schools. After all, a school that holds little store by pastoral care is surely not one you would wish your child to attend.

We have found that the majority of problems with teachers are more likely to occur when the child goes to secondary school and pupils are considered old enough to be responsible for themselves. This is a fair enough attitude, and one that will help them make the transition to an independent life. You also have to remember that the schools are bigger and the teachers are under more pressure to get their pupils through GCSEs and A levels. So, if your child is not yet at secondary school, be prepared for this change and, unless there is any real reason to feel that staff are being *deliberately* unhelpful, you should not feel offended.

As far as bunking school goes, many adolescents play truant from class or skip a full day once in a while. To a certain extent, all teenagers go through phases of resenting the fact that they are obliged to attend school and sit through dull lessons that seem to bear little relevance to life as they know it. Be honest, did you never *ever* take a day off 'sick'? However, truanting more than, say, once a term and not feeling guilty about it can quickly escalate and become a real issue.

If your teenager is either using his diabetes as an excuse not to go to school (feigning hypos and other assorted symptoms), leaving the house but not arriving at school or blatantly refusing to go to school, then you need to find out why. The other truants he may be mixing with could spell trouble as, spending days sitting around doing nothing leads to boredom and this can lead to delinquency and drug-taking. But if, as in Tom's case, the problem does seem to be diabetes-related, you need help from both his diabetes team and the school as soon as possible, so things may be sorted out before he really digs himself into a hole.

If the problem has less to do with diabetes than his belief that school is a waste of time and the headteacher has reached the end of their tether, then a family therapist could help you handle the situation before it falls into the hands of the Social Services (which long-term absenteeism from school invariably does).

All our teenagers agreed that they appreciated a low-key approach to their diabetes at school, being able to keep hypo-stoppers in their blazer pockets or school bags without having to trek to a first aid cupboard if they needed glucose or having to explain to a teacher why they were munching glucose tablets in the middle of a lesson. They didn't want dinner ladies tut-tutting when they helped themselves to pudding or PE staff repeatedly asking them if they had taken their snack before exercise. They valued explanations about diabetes to the class, but in the context of a biology or PSE class rather than have the finger pointing directly at themselves. They were happy to give talks on diabetes, do projects on diabetes, organize sponsored swims and so on for diabetes, but mainly if this was in a 'special interest' context. As far as day-to-day living was concerned, they didn't want special attention and certainly no pity. As Debbie said:

> *There's nothing to be embarrassed about and you shouldn't try and make people feel sorry for you or you won't get any respect.*

Fortunately, however, most of the young people who responded to our survey coped happily with their friend's interest in the condition. Gareth, 15, reported:

> *All my friends know I have diabetes. One of them is even doing a section on diabetes and sport for his GCSE coursework thanks to me!*

When Vanessa's diabetes equipment went missing from the bathroom at her boarding school, 'the entire school dropped everything . . . every single person looked for the stuff, even in the dustbins. They were wonderful.'

Many parents felt strongly that schools should educate pupils on various chronic conditions such as diabetes, asthma, eczema, epilepsy and so on as a matter of course. One father, Robert, put it bluntly:

Some sort of proper information should be available at school to help educate the few idiots that take the mick, as this can be very hurtful.

Driving Matters

Most young people approaching 17 can't wait to learn to drive. Your teenager may not realize that there are certain requirements that he must be able to fulfil in order to be granted a licence. On application for a licence, the form will ask the standard questions, including whether you have now or ever had any of a number of medical problems. Your teenager must, by law, answer 'yes' to the question relating to diabetes and must state whether his diabetes is controlled by insulin or tablets. After the application form has been returned to the Driver and Vehicle Licensing Agency (DVLA), he will be sent a supplementary form (Diabetic 1), which asks for further information and the address of his GP and/or hospital doctor. He will also be asked to sign a consent form so that the DVLA can contact his doctor directly if necessary.

If all this is new information to your teenager, expect some ranting and raving about how unfair it is to be singled out and possibly denied a licence because of his diabetes. Point out that, yes, *life* is unfair because he happens to have diabetes, but that it's not unreasonable for the DVLA to be questioning how fit he is to be out on the road and that all this boils down to his diabetes control.

The DVLA itself points out that it wishes to issue licences, not refuse them or take them away, but that it needs to receive honest and relevant information regarding the state of your teenager's health in order to ensure that he is not a hazard on the road, that is, having hypos at the wheel and endangering the lives of others (and his own).

The information given to the DVLA by the doctor will state how well controlled the youngster's diabetes is and this may well be the motivation he needs to strive for good control (if he has been badly controlled until now). There are questions about hypoglycaemia in general. If he has been admitted to hospital following a severe hypo, then the licence may not be issued for up until six months have passed without a hospital admission. Essentially, your teenager should not be driving if:

- he is being stabilized on insulin – until stabilization is complete
- he has difficulty in recognizing the early symptoms of hypos, which may lead to aggressive behaviour, poor muscle control and even sudden unconsciousness, all of which should not happen while he is at the wheel
- he has any problems with his eyesight that cannot be corrected by glasses
- he has numbness or weakness in the hands or feet due to diabetic neuropathy
- his control is poor and has necessitated hospital admissions for hypos or he has to be constantly assisted while hypo.

If none of the above conditions apply and the doctor confirms that there are no complications that might impair your teenager's safety as a driver, then there is no reason for him not to be granted a licence.

A person with insulin-dependent diabetes will be issued a licence for one, two or three years and renewals (for which reminders will be sent automatically) will be made free of charge. Provisional licences are also restricted to one, two and three years. If any changes in treatment occur or problems develop that may affect the youngster's ability to drive, he must inform the DVLA. If the teenager was diagnosed as having diabetes *after* obtaining his licence, he must, by law, inform the DVLA, which will then send him the necessary forms for further information.

Judy (now 23) admits to feeling angry and bitter when her licence application was initially turned down:

I knew that my control left a lot to be desired . . . I'd ended up in hospital three times in eight months and I got a flat refusal. In fact, it was the making of me because I took myself in hand, my control became really good quite quickly, but I didn't even think about applying again for some time. This time, there was no question of

101

refusal. I've been driving for three years and my licence has been renewed every year.

Debbie was somewhat taken aback when she told her driving instructor that she had diabetes:

He replied that he should have been able to tell by looking at my eyes! There's not much you can say to that, is there?

Insurance is a big bone of contention for many drivers who have diabetes. By law, every driver must be insured against the risk of liability for injury to third parties. Most insurers will offer cover to people with diabetes, but, in some circumstances, charge a higher premium. This loading, coupled with the fact that those under 25 pay higher premiums anyway, can make the cost of insurance prohibitive. In fact, if your teenager's diabetes is well-controlled and stable, he should not have problems in obtaining cover at normal rates, so the answer is to shop around and obtain quotes from several different companies or else use a good broker who will do the groundwork and should be able to obtain the best deal.

The BDA receives many complaints about discrimination from insurance companies and suggests these are challenged. However, it has negotiated competitively priced exclusive schemes for people with diabetes (motoring, life and travel insurance) so it's worth contacting the BDA for information about these.

Make sure your teenager is aware that he *must* tell the insurers he has diabetes. If this information is withheld and he is then involved in an accident, the insurers are likely to dismiss any claim by making the policy null and void on the grounds of non-disclosure.

Although certain restrictions do make sense, we tend to agree with those who complain that insurance companies can be petty and nit-picking, as one mother, Pat, found out:

When Lynn started taking driving lessons, I could not get her included on my insurance until she passed her test. She resented this very much. I tried other companies but they were just the same. However, there's been no problem since she passed. As Lynn's diabetes control is extremely good (and was at that time) why should she have been treated differently to any other learner driver who can be put on her parent's insurance?

Your teenager should remember that if he has an accident while hypo, he could well be charged with dangerous or careless driving or driving under the influence of a drug (although, in 1957, a motorist with diabetes once argued with the High Court that insulin in law is a hormone and not actually a drug, but this was overruled). In this case, the youngster's licence could be taken away, unless he appeals successfully that the hypo was due to unusual circumstances and is unlikely to happen again. But, even so, his insurance premiums would certainly increase after such an incident. So, as a matter of course, the following rules should always apply to your teenager when driving:

- always carry some form of glucose and keep glucose tablets, chocolate, sandwiches or biscuits in the car
- make sure some carbohydrate has been eaten before embarking on a journey, however short
- never drive for more than two hours without stopping for a snack
- never drive if meals have been delayed or missed
- keep spare blood test equipment in the car and test before and, if necessary, during a journey to make sure blood glucose levels are satisfactory
- if the early symptoms of a hypo are felt, stop driving immediately and do not start again until the symptoms have disappeared completely and make it clear that you are no longer in charge of the car by removing the ignition key and either getting out of the car or moving across to the passenger seat so there can be no suggestion that you are in charge of a car while under the influence of drugs
- never drink and drive – this, of course, applies to every motorist, but, if you are on insulin, a hypo may appear to be

drunkenness and if your breath smells of alcohol, suspicions will be increased (incidentally, contrary to some beliefs, the presence of ketones on the breath will not register a false positive on a breathalyser machine).

Do reiterate to your teenager that the laws on diabetes and driving are not unfair (unless, of course, he is refused a licence even though he has fulfilled all the medical requirements, in which case he should contact the BDA for help and advice). Try to make him appreciate that if his safety (and the safety of others) is in question, then it is only right that he is prohibited from driving. However, good blood glucose control is inevitably the answer and this should be an incentive for him to get into shape for now and the future.

Work Worries

To quote from the *Diabetes Employment Handbook* (BDA, London, 1992):

> *Despite recent advances in the control of diabetes, the condition is still feared and misunderstood by some employers. This can resultin difficulty and discrimination both for those with diabetes who are seeking employment and those who are already employed.*

Of course, thousands of people with insulin-dependent diabetes have good careers or jobs that they enjoy, but that doesn't mean to say that it's been an easy ride in all cases, and there are many stories of disappointment along the way with some rather nonsensical rules to boot. Seventeen-year-old Susie asks:

> *Why is it that a policeman who develops diabetes during his career can keep his job and yet someone who has diabetes and applies for a job with the police will definitely be turned down? It's annoying that diabetes restricts me from having certain jobs . . . Personally I would*

not like to do any of them anyway, but there are probably lots of people who would.

Andrew, 16, agrees:

I will not be able to join the police force, which had always been my choice of a future career. I think this is quite ridiculous as they let in heavy smokers and drinkers with probably poorer health than myself.

One mother was understandably indignant for her 17-year-old son:

The realization that diabetes can cause trouble with work hit us last year when Gary applied for a job at Shell Oil. It took six months from start to finish, with the conclusion being that Gary could not work offshore because he had insulin-dependent diabetes. The quite extraordinary part is that he was applying for onshore *work and they* knew *he had diabetes. He got to the stage of signing a conditional contract after having successfully completed two interviews, the condition being that he had to pass a medical. It was after the medical that Gary was considered unfit for offshore work . . . which he had never applied for in the first place!*

It is cases such as Gary's that are distasteful and, frankly, ridiculous. There are so many similar cases of such discrimination that a whole book could be written on this subject alone. However, the BDA fights hard to win appeals for those who come up against such discrimination and, for example, at the time of writing, it was in discussion with the Home Office regarding guidelines for fire-fighting. A number of appeals had been successful and the BDA aims to change the nature of prejudiced assessments in many fields. Unless there is a clear guideline as to why your son or daughter's diabetes should prevent him or her from doing a particular job, then it is certainly worth contacting the BDA for help and advice.

In many careers – such as journalism, law, medicine, banking, the computer industry, teaching and broadcasting – the applicant is open to individual assessment, the results of which will probably be based on medical information from your child's doctor. Happily, the majority of working teenagers in our survey had jobs that they enjoyed and had not encountered problems. Good blood glucose control, regular attendance at work and no suggestion of diabetes interfering with the job in hand led to successful employment.

Katy, a veterinary nurse, told us:

I was given a real grilling over my ability to work the long hours, but I answered all the questions with conviction. I got the job . . . it was hard at first, remembering to eat when things were so busy, but I've been there two years now and I love it.

Roger – now in his thirties – felt that having diabetes actually *helped* when he went for his first job as a dentist:

Maybe they thought my having a medical condition would help me have a more personal touch with the patients. I don't know whether that's true in dentistry, but I'm sure it is in, say, medicine and nursing.

Unfortunately, it's a fact that there remain many who are forced to rethink their original choice of career. For instance, at the time of writing, there was a blanket ban on those with insulin-dependent diabetes entering the armed forces, the police, diving, air crews (private or commercial), driving trains, buses or HGV lorries.

However concerned you may feel reading this, you have to put it all into perspective and remember that many, many top professionals, sports personalities, actors, creative people and all kinds of other members of the workforce have diabetes. But, we do reiterate that any seemingly unfair discrimination should be challenged, not only for your own youngster, but for the sake of others.

It's interesting that statistics show that children with diabetes frequently have a better record of attendance than their non-diabetic counterparts and often fare better than average in exams.

Maybe they are conscious of proving that they are just as normal as everyone else and, although there are no similar statistics available for working people with diabetes, surely it follows that the same attitude should prevail later in life?

Chapter 8

SEX, DRUGS AND ROCK 'N' ROLL

The title of this chapter may be a well-worn cliché, but it best sums up the excesses of the teenage generation that parents fear most. We've all been teenagers ourselves and, to a greater or lesser extent, had cause to turn our own parents into nervous wrecks. Yet, it seems today that our children grow up faster and experiment with potential dangers earlier than we did, simply because so much more is openly discussed and easily available to them. We might not want to face up to the fact that our sons or daughters have under-age sex or are able to buy drugs in the school playground, but the possibility is there and no parent should imagine that their offspring is immune. As a parent of a teenager with diabetes, you need as much information as possible to help you understand and cope if your child does seem to be going off the rails.

Sex and the Teenage Girl

Compared to other European countries, sex education in Britain is considered to be poor and the rate of births to 15- to 19-year-old mothers is the highest. In the UK, the pregnancy rate is 65 per 1,000. A staggering 8,000 girls under the age of consent have babies each year and the teenage abortion rate is five times higher than that of the Dutch, who place a lot of value on sex education.

There have always been risks associated with diabetes in pregnancy, but these have greatly decreased over the years as understanding of the condition has led to the realization that tight control of blood glucose levels even before conception goes a long way towards producing a normal, healthy baby. Home blood testing and better diabetes counselling at the preconception stage now mean that the statistics for healthy babies born to mothers with diabetes are virtually the same as those for mothers who do not have diabetes. This is a huge improvement on the 1950s, when 25 per cent of women with diabetes in the UK lost their babies through miscarriage or stillbirth and many more babies were born with defects such as spina bifida, heart problems or missing fingers or toes. Pregnant women with poorly controlled diabetes do still run the risk of having big babies, as glucose from the mother crosses the placenta to the baby. This in turn stimulates the baby to produce larger amounts of insulin. The mechanism by which insulin stimulates foetal growth is not yet clear but for some reason, maybe because of the stimulation of growth hormone, the baby grows very large. This 'macrosomic' (large) baby can produce all sorts of problems during and after the birth. For example, a big baby can induce premature labour, there is a greater risk of needing to have the baby by Caesarian section, and the baby's lungs may be immature so the baby would need to go in to a special care baby unit after birth.

So, with this latter information in mind, it is easy to see how an *unplanned* pregnancy could have a devastating outcome for a teenage girl with diabetes, and, indeed, the whole family. Without wishing to scare the living daylights out of your daughter, it is important that she understands the possible consequences of an unplanned diabetic pregnancy. However, she should be fully informed, on the positive side, that when she is ready to have children, looking after herself before conception and during pregnancy bring very high chances of success. Help is available to her, as a great number of hospitals and clinics run prepregnancy counselling services.

All this, of course, is information for the future, but your daughter should certainly be aware of the facts. If you feel unable to talk to her on this subject, have a quiet word with your diabetes nurse or doctor to make sure someone explains this to her. So, for the above reasons, you can see that once your daughter starts being sexually active she needs to know all about contraception.

You may not like to face up to it, but teenagers these days tend to become sexually active at an earlier age than did those of their parent's generation. One recent survey in a teenage magazine showed that over 50 per cent of girls interviewed had first experienced intercourse aged 14 or 15 – some as young as 13. All kinds of theories abound as to why this should be, yet, if this is the case with your daughter, all that matters now is that she is protected from unwanted pregnancy and sexually transmitted diseases. This, of course, is where sex education in schools is so important, but whether or not your child's school provides it adequately is hit and miss. Some schools provide excellent guidance, some considerably less – so you need to find out how much your daughter really understands about birth control. The Brook Advisory Centres (see the Useful Addresses section at the back of this book) are excellent at helping and advising teenagers – with or without mum in tow – or your GP could offer advice.

Below, the methods of contraception most suitable for teenage girls are described – and, remember that having diabetes does not mean your daughter is any less fertile than a non-diabetic woman, so if your daughter is sexually active, then contraception is a priority. Incidentally, although the same risks are obviously not applicable to boys, they should also be aware of acting responsibly and using condoms *every* time they have intercourse.

Suitable Forms of Contraception

Oral Contraceptives
THE PILL: The combined pill is so called because it combines two hormones – progesterone and oestrogen. The levels of oestrogen they contain these days are far lower than in the original Pills of the 1960s and 1970s, which has considerably lessened the number of

side-effects they have. Consult your doctor if you have any concerns about the recent publicity surrounding the third generation Pill.

This type of Pill may require an alteration to be made to insulin levels, although this would be small. If there is a family history of heart attacks or stroke, though, then this type of Pill should be avoided and it is not recommended for smokers (smoking when you have diabetes is bad news anyway, as described below).

If it is suitable for your daughter, the combined pill is an effective method of contraception. However, the majority of doctors prefer not to prescribe the Pill to younger teenagers (those below the age of 15).

The mini pill contains progesterone only and, because of this, it is not as effective as the combined pill. However, it can be used by women who have a family history of heart disease and stroke. For maximum effect, this Pill should be taken strictly at the same time of day, perhaps with the evening insulin. It has to be remembered that most teenagers are not reliable when it comes to sticking to rigid times and this should be seriously taken into consideration.

Both the combined and mini pills can be rendered ineffective by certain antibiotics, some drugs, diarrhoea and vomiting. If your daughter is prescribed any new medication, for whatever reason, then she should tell the doctor that she is taking the Pill and she should use an additional method of contraception, such as a condom.

Barrier Methods

Condoms, or sheaths, are probably the form of contraception your teenager will be most familiar with. Advertisements for condoms are common and many public toilets have condom machines.

When used correctly (and in conjunction with a spermicidal jelly or cream), they are certainly as effective as the mini pill. Unfortunately, they are not always put on properly, so if your teenager is going to be using condoms, it would be a good idea for her (or him) to see a family planning nurse, to be sure how a condom should be used.

As well as protecting against pregnancy, condoms also help prevent the spread of sexually transmitted diseases, including HIV and AIDS. Female condoms (Femidom) are available, and girls can also use a diaphragm (cap), which can be fitted by her GP or at the family planning clinic. It really is advisable to use a spermicidal jelly or cream with any barrier method.

Norplant

Under local anaesthetic, six flexible, matchstick-size rods containing the hormone levonorgestrol are inserted under the skin of the inside upper arm. They release the hormone into the bloodstream to prevent pregnancy.

The implant stays in place for five years (although it can be removed at any time) and, once removed, fertility is not affected. Side-effects can include lighter periods and irregular bleeding. Also, some women have had considerable problems with having the implants removed.

IUDs

These letters stand for intra-uterine devices, and these are commonly called the coil. They are not recommended for teenage women (particularly those with diabetes) as there is a risk of pelvic inflammatory disease, which can lead to infertility.

Emergency Contraception

Your daughter should also know about the 'morning after pill', which can be taken up to 72 hours after intercourse, whether unprotected or if, for instance, a condom has torn.

The Rhythm Method

This involves avoiding intercourse at the time of ovulation and is the least effective method of contraception as the teenage cycle can be erratic and poorly controlled. Diabetes is likely to make this worse. Not recommended.

Sex and Hypos

Sex is a form of exercise and, as with all forms of exercise, hypos can be a problem if steps are not taken to prevent glucose levels falling too low. Of course, a hypo during sex can be a real embarrassment to some teenagers – interrupting a moment of passion to munch glucose tablets is hardly romantic! However, if they *don't* reach for the hypostoppers, it might be far more embarrassing to become incoherent and need assistance!

With some forms of exercise, the teenager is able to plan what to do about insulin or food, but, of course, sex tends to be more spontaneous. The best thing is to keep hypostoppers at hand just in case. Having a sugary drink is probably the simplest solution. Also as with any other form of exercise, a hypo can occur after sex, so having a snack afterwards will help ward this off.

It is important that your teenager discusses diabetes and hypos with her partner so everything is out in the open. Maybe embarrassment is best avoided by making light of the matter, as Jackie, 19, remembers:

> *I had to ask my boyfriend to stop so I could get some sugar. To get over the embarrassment I told him it was the amazing effect he was having on me. That really boosted his ego!*

If you find it difficult to talk about sex with your teenager, don't bury your head in the sand and assume she or he will learn all about it 'sometime' – that may be too late. You can contact their diabetes nurse or family planning clinic (ask for the nearest clinic at your GP's surgery) and a chat with her or him can be arranged without your having to be involved.

Smoking, Drinking and Drugs

Smoking

Tobacco is a stimulant and contains nicotine, which is a drug and can be addictive. Although it is illegal to sell cigarettes and loose tobacco to children under 16, many shopkeepers unfortunately ignore this law and the kids soon find out who will sell them cigarettes (often singly when they can't afford a packet). However, it is not actually illegal for children to smoke and a survey carried out in 1990 found that 25 per cent of girls and 25 per cent of boys who responded were regular smokers by the age of 15.

Smokers know that what they are doing is bad for them and increases the risks of coronary and lung diseases, but as people with diabetes are more prone to heart attacks, stroke and circulatory problems anyway, they should understand why smoking is an even bigger risk for them – a complete no-no.

It was encouraging to discover that the vast majority of teenagers in our survey did not smoke and had not been tempted to start, saying things like:

It's a disgusting smelly habit.

I've never tried it and the thought of it makes me feel sick.

I didn't smoke before I developed diabetes and I'm certainly not about to now.

I admit that I used to smoke and it's taken me a long time to give up. But, I've done it and I have to admit I feel much better for it.

But what can you do if your teenager *does* smoke?

Your own attitude towards smoking plays an important part in whether or not your child smokes. If there are smokers in your household, then your child is twice as likely to follow suit. If your teenager knows you disapprove, then she may be less likely to smoke, but going on about it endlessly can make her rebel and start.

Peer pressure is the usual cause of most youngsters starting smoking, and if this is the case then you must point out that smoking and diabetes do not mix. Also, make the case that stale smoke lingers in clothing, in hair and on the breath. It is ageing, as lines develop around the lips from 'dragging' on cigarettes and the skin ages prematurely. Appealing to her sense of vanity may help, as may adding that smoking is expensive and surely her money could be put to better use! However, constant nagging and tantrums are likely to have the opposite effect to the one desired. Point out the facts calmly but firmly – smoking will do her no favours and is likely to harm her a great deal.

Drinking

On average, men consume about 8 pints of beer a week and women the equivalent of 3 pints, but it's a fact that young adults (in their late teens and early twenties) drink more than the average. It is illegal for those under 18 to buy or consume alcohol on licensed premises, although there are always publicans who turn a blind eye. To be fair, some teenagers do look older than they really are and, without asking for ID, it can be hard to make correct judgements.

The main reason for drinking alcohol is that it makes people feel relaxed, and many say it helps their confidence. However, drinking to excess can cause slurred speech, unsteadiness, double vision, vomiting and, eventually, loss of consciousness, not to mention road accidents, violence and all kinds of household dangers, such as fires. It's also true that young adults are more susceptible to the effects of alcohol than older people, so the key to drinking is moderation.

As we discussed in Chapter 4, there is no reason for those with diabetes not to drink, so long as they take it easy. Older teenagers who are likely to drink should know the rules. As we also stressed in Chapter 4, alcohol-related hypos can be a real danger.

But, once again, your attitude towards alcohol will influence your child. If you are perceived to be a heavy drinker, then your son or daughter may think nothing of knocking back several drinks a night (and it's usually boys who are the culprits here). Try to set an example for your child to follow and be sure to get the message across to your teenager that if a drinking session is on the cards, then she must have something to eat before or at the party, pub or wherever she is going. Remind her to take hypostoppers and diabetes ID. From then on, she is responsible for herself as you must assume – rightly or wrongly – that her friends will be drinking as well and may not notice if she has a hypo.

Drugs and Solvent Abuse

All kinds of drugs are available to today's teenagers, who are generally pretty knowledgeable about them as they can find out all kinds of information from every part of the media. Indeed, they often hear about it first-hand from older adolescents who have experimented with drugs themselves. Don't fool yourself, *any* child can become involved with drugs. Drugs may be offered to youngsters wherever they may be.

Young people seldom think of the consequences of becoming addicted to drugs. They want to experiment and cannot imagine that they could ruin their lives if a harmless buzz turned into a dangerous habit. Many of today's teenagers will have had their first puff of a joint by the age of 13 and, from there on, a pattern will follow as to whether they take drugs socially (for reasons similar to those for social drinking) or sample stronger and more addictive drugs as a habit. Some teenagers are not interested in becoming involved at all in the first place. We were surprised and delighted with the majority of comments teenagers made in our survey:

A lot of people I know smoke pot. I don't really mind unless they do it excessively, which I think is stupid. I don't have the desire (or enough money!) to do recreational drugs. Even if I had the money, I wouldn't.

I think it's OK to do them as long as you're in control, but this is often not the case. I've smoked pot, but not often enough to be a regular buyer. Effects as far as diabetes is concerned . . . ? Probably better to deal with than drink. I do eat more as it lowers blood glucose levels. I've also done a 'trip' and 'speed' but these seemed to have no effect on my diabetes at all. I only did these once to see what they were like and I don't have any intention of doing them again, even though I suffered no ill-effects.

I think people who use drugs to get a buzz are stupid . . . but if they want to risk their lives, let them.

Barbara, mother of 19-year-old Mark, said:

Drug pushers and drug-taking in general anger Mark greatly since he is forced to inject to stay alive. He can't understand people willingly abusing their bodies simply for kicks. He enjoys raves, but he goes to forget his problems and dance all night, not take drugs.

As a parent, you need to be able to give your child the right information on drugs and you will earn their respect by appearing knowledgeable on a subject that they assume is only understood by their peers. Below is a basic guide to drugs and solvents. We have outlined their effects on diabetes, but the most common problem is the user becoming high and then hypo because they forget to eat. The chances are, too, that her friends will also be high and not notice the state she is in.

Amphetamines

In the 1960s, these drugs were used to treat depression and widely used as appetite suppressants for would-be slimmers. Today, they can be bought as powder, capsules or pills. Amphetamines, or speed, can be injected and even smoked and the powder can also be snorted up the nose.

The drug is actually a stimulant (ecstasy is derived from it), but can cause panic attacks, anxiety and insomnia. High doses can produce hallucinations, delirium and dehydration. There is always the risk of HIV infection and hepatitis with shared needles if the user injects amphetamine.

The hyperactive effect produced by speed can also be

dangerous to those with heart or blood pressure problems. Because the appetite is suppressed, the danger to someone with diabetes is that they will not bother to eat, even if they are aware that they should, causing hypos, which the stimulant properties of the drug will exacerbate. Once the effect of speed wears off, the user will be starving hungry and probably overeat to compensate, so blood glucose levels will be going haywire.

Cannabis

The most widely used illegal drug in the UK, it is also referred to as pot, marijuana, hash, grass or dope (among other names) and comes from the *Cannabis sativa* plant. Herbal cannabis can be smoked by itself, but is more usually mixed with tobacco in a roll-up cigarette or pipe. The resin can be smoked and is sometimes eaten or added to dishes such as cakes (hash brownies).

The effects depend on the user's mood, but, usually, it helps people to relax, making them giggly, uninhibited and enhancing their appreciation of music, sounds and colour. If the drug is taken while depressed or anxious, though, then these feelings may be heightened. Cannabis affects concentration and the effects start soon after taking (when smoking) and can last for several hours.

Although not a physically addictive drug as such, psychological dependence can occur – as is the case with other non-addictive drugs. Also, long-term heavy smoking may lead to lung disorders and the effect of cannabis itself as a carcinogenic substance has been suggested. Although in theory cannabis could help settle blood glucose because of its relaxing properties, the risk of hypos while stoned outweighs this. As cannabis affects concentration and sometimes the ability to carry out simple tasks, your teenager may forget to eat and not recognize or be able to react to having a hypo.

Cocaine and Crack

Cocaine, or coke, is derived from the South American coca shrub and is refined into a powder, which is usually snorted through a makeshift tube, such as a rolled-up banknote or a straw. Sometimes it is injected from a solution. A line of coke is a prepared line ready for snorting.

Crack (also known as ice or rock) is cocaine that has been treated with chemicals, so it is cheaper as it is not pure. Crack is smoked in a pipe, plastic bottle, glass tube or on foil. Users inhale the smoke from the heated rocks.

Cocaine and crack stimulate the central nervous system, making users feel elated, strong, often sexually powerful and sometimes violent. The effects come quickly, but end suddenly and the dose needs repeating about every 20 minutes to maintain the high. Regular use is less to do with actual physical dependence than the psychological need for repeated hits to keep the effects going. Continued use increases the risk of abnormal heart rhythms, high blood pressure, convulsions, heart attack and heart failure.

Cocaine is safer (if that's an appropriate word!) than crack because it is in a pure form. However, at £50 a gram, its cost is prohibitive to many would-be users who are able to obtain crack far more cheaply. In fact, the use of cocaine and crack in this country is far less common than the media might have us believe, unlike in the United States where it has been described as an epidemic. Again, the risk of going into a hypo while high is ever present.

Ecstasy

This is a 'designer' drug derived from amphetamines. It is also known as E, MDMA, disco biscuits or doves. It comes in tablet form (white or brown) or a variety of differently coloured capsules.

The effect E produces starts about 20 minutes after it has been taken and can last for hours. It tends to make people extra-sociable and heightens the perception of sound and colour. It can also cause users to become uncoordinated and confused. Taken regularly over several days, the user may suffer from insomnia or paranoia. Once the effect has worn off, it can leave the user feeling very depressed and down.

In the long term, users build up a tolerance to E, which means they will need to take more and more for the required effect or move on to try something else to get their buzz.

There have been widely publicized cases of deaths caused by reactions to this drug (which sometimes is because what was taken was a mixture of chemicals and not pure), as well as breathing problems, heart failure, kidney and liver damage. Some research suggests it can also cause brain damage.

E is often taken at raves, which involve all-night frenetic dancing. Alcohol is nearly always banned from these events (thankfully), but drinking liquids is essential to prevent dehydration. Hypos can be a real risk at raves (see later in this chapter) and, as long-term use of E causes liver damage, having a hypo once this has happened could be extremely dangerous, as damage to the liver may prevent the release of stored glucose, the mechanism that normally brings someone with diabetes out of a hypo. As E also causes kidney damage, this will hasten kidney failure in people with diabetes who already have some degree of nephropathy

Heroin

Heroin is an opiate, a pain-killing drug. It is a powder derived from the opium poppy. It is also known as smack, dragon, junk and gear. Heroin can be smoked, snorted or injected and is highly physically addictive.

It is often mixed with other drugs, but sometimes with glucose, giving users a feeling of warmth and drowsiness and relaxed detachment from emotional or physical pain. Those who are not used to it can have bad experiences, including nausea and vomiting. Tolerance develops with regular use, so more and more is needed to obtain the desired effect. Users do not pay much attention to their health and their diet is often poor. Also, the risk of blood-borne infections, such as HIV and hepatitis, is high. Physical withdrawal after regular use is highly unpleasant and usually requires specialized medical help as the psychological and physical need for the drug is often desperate.

Someone who is high on heroin could be mistaken for being hypo as the symptoms are similar – those of slurred speech and drowsiness. As dietary intake is poor, there is an extreme risk of a hypo, although, conversely, a regular heroin user may not bother or may forget to inject insulin altogether, thus risking hyperglycaemic coma.

LSD

Famous for its hallucinogenic or psychedelic properties back in the 1960s, LSD, or acid (from its chemical name, lysergic acid diethylamide), has made something of a comeback on today's drug scene. LSD comes in tablet or capsule form ('a tab of acid') and paper and sugar cubes can be impregnated with the drug.

The effects of LSD largely depend on the mood the user is in at the time and, to some extent, who she is with. A trip can last for up to 12 hours and can be exciting, intensely self-exploratory, with heightened awareness of sight and sound and changes in sense of time and place, as well as feelings of being outside yourself. However, a bad trip can be extremely disturbing, with terrifying hallucinations, paranoia, dizziness and suicidal despair.

LSD tends to be used on an occasional basis as a 'special' recreational drug. There is no known physical risk from long-term use unless a bad trip is experienced when the user could endanger her own life. Eating is hardly going to be a priority when on a psychedelic trip and the danger of unnoticed hypos is a very real one.

Magic Mushrooms

These are wild mushrooms that have hallucinogenic properties. The main type is the liberty cap (*Psilocybe*) and they are often referred to as liberties. Picking and eating the mushrooms raw is not illegal, but, once they are cooked, dried or made into a preparation to be used as a hallucinogen they then become illegal.

The effect of magic mushrooms depends on the user and the situation in which they are taking the drug. High doses can give a mild trip with colour and sound distortions, but a bad trip can be frightening and include nausea and vomiting – particularly dangerous if the user has diabetes. Unrecognized hypos are, of course, also a problem. The other real danger is that the wrong mushrooms could be picked and many mushrooms are poisonous.

Solvents

After smoking and alcohol, solvents are the substances young people are most likely to try because they are easy to obtain. One in ten secondary school children (the peak age is around 13 or 14) try sniffing solvents, although, thankfully, most only experiment. There is a wide range of products that can be used, including aerosol sprays, butane gas, glue and correcting fluids. Aerosols and butane gas can be sniffed from plastic bags, can lids or by spraying directly into the mouth. Glue is also sniffed from bags.

The effects of sniffing can be similar to those of alcohol, but the buzz happens more quickly as the solvent is absorbed into the bloodstream from the lungs.

Solvent abuse is highly dangerous as the breathing and heart rate are lowered. There is also the risk of suffocation from aerosols or plastic bags, and butane gas may ignite in the mouth. Some teenagers are more susceptible to the harmful effects than others and permanent damage may be caused, sometimes death.

Solvent abusers often forget to eat or do not want to. A child with diabetes may not bother to inject insulin at all and the consequences can be catastrophic.

Solvent abusers tend to prefer being on their own, in out-of-the-way places, but even if the teenager were with other misusers, they would be unlikely to notice if she were hypo or hyper. The majority of youngsters who experiment with solvents are highly unlikely to become regular users. Keep an eye out for empty aerosol cans or glue containers in your child's room and be aware of any chemical-based smells.

How to Handle the Subject

Drug-taking is not rife among the majority of young people, but temptation is often there and teenagers are usually curious to experiment. Even if they *try* drugs, it doesn't mean they are on the road to addiction or regular drug-taking. Most youngsters lose interest or form the opinion that it's unhealthy and a waste of time, while some use them occasionally and seem to be in control.

However, if you suspect that your child really does have a problem and uses drugs regularly, there are certain signs to look for. Remember, though, that many of these symptoms are quite normal adolescent behaviour, so don't jump in at the deep end before you have the full story. There is a new kit on the market that enables parents to test a suspected drug-user's room for various substances, but the general feeling is that this could make the situation worse as the teenager would see this as a betrayal of trust and privacy. Communication and awareness are better methods of detection, but here are some of the signs to watch out for:

- marked swings of mood, restlessness, aggression
- noticeable decline in standards of schoolwork
- bunking school
- furtive behaviour and unwillingness to introduce you to new friends
- stealing money, jewellery and so on
- lack of appetite (poor blood glucose control and unwillingness to do blood tests)
- excessive tiredness and apathy
- sores or rashes around the nose or mouth
- interest in drug paraphernalia, noticing shredded cigarettes, torn cigarette packets or pieces of card, aerosols, lighter fuel cans, glue pots scattered around the teenager's bedroom
- unusual smells in the house or stains on the clothes.

Please remember that it's important not to jump to conclusions too quickly, but if you really do suspect – or find out – that your teenager is taking drugs, then it will certainly help to talk to someone who specializes in this area (see your phone book for drug helplines).

As we have tried to stress throughout this book, going on and on about something will just end in arguments and usually have the opposite effect to the one you want. Try to deal with the matter in hand calmly and seek professional advice if necessary.

Rock 'n' Roll (and Other Social Activities)

Teenagers want to be independent and have a hectic social life – without you breathing down their necks and worrying. You may be getting het up over a rave, an all-night party or even a camping trip with the Girl Guides – all different types of social fun for your youngster, but all sounding warning bells in your head as far as her diabetes is concerned.

The activities you will be concerned about probably involve extra exercise and the possibility of hypos. Camping may *sound* innocuous, but who's to say that a hike won't take three times longer than expected? Raves have had a bad press, but they are really today's equivalent of discos, and the disastrous illegal raves we've heard about in disused warehouses and fields are largely out of fashion now. Many teenagers go to 'official' raves, which often take place in leisure or community centres and are organized and advertised properly. Participants are searched for drugs on entry and alcohol is banned. Other raves are not so particular about drugs and these are more likely to be held in clubs. Even so, alcohol is not allowed and fizzy drinks, orange juice or mineral water is usually on sale. If you have expressed your concerns and she has agreed to eat beforehand, drink sugary drinks to keep up her glucose levels with all the dancing and phone you during the evening, then let her go and hope for the best. After all, her motives for going to a rave will not be to discover drugs – if that's all she's interested in she will already have done that! Incidentally, some youngsters take their own drinks to raves, although this is not allowed in some establishments. Your teenager should always carry glucose tablets in case water is all that can be obtained.

The best advice you can instil in your teenager is 'be prepared'. Wherever she's going, whatever she's doing, try to get her to be forearmed should problems arise. Jenny says:

> *I feel sad that I can't be as spontaneous as my friends, but I do every-thing that I can to keep up without putting myself in danger. I eat before I go out, take glucose tablets and money for extra food, insulin just in case I'm invited to stay at a friends and I wear ID in case any-thing goes wrong. I have to think ahead – very fast sometimes – which I'd rather not do . . . But I can't say I miss out on anything.*

Whatever your teenager is planning to do, whether it's a rave, sleepover party, sports tournament or camping trip, spell out the rules:

- food – eat carbohydrates regularly and keep extra money for emergencies
- wear ID at all times
- take hypostoppers to cover any eventuality, such as not being able to get food on time or there being no suitable drinks at raves or parties
- make sure she tells you where she's going, who she's going with and insist that you're informed if the plan changes
- tell her you'd like a phonecall – many teenagers carry phonecards or the special BT cards that can be programmed to connect with their home number only
- she should take her insulin (and blood test kit ideally) if she's staying over at a friend's house
- make sure her friends know she has diabetes and how to cope in an emergency – assure her that they would far rather know than be completely in the dark should she have a hypo, and appeal to her sense of loyalty by explaining that *not* telling them would make them feel really stupid if they were unable to help.

Of course you're going to be worried despite such preparation, but you have to remember that teenagers in general *are* a worry – diabetes or not. It's also true, though, that most of them come out the other side unscathed and perfectly responsible adults. Didn't you? Don't let the fact that your teenager has diabetes spoil this time of growing up. Just help her to understand and appreciate that you've only got her best interests at heart, and you can help her to realize that diabetes can become not so much a problem, more a way of life. By putting some thought into a situation, the fun does not have to be spoiled. As Tim says:

> *Compensate for what you're doing beforehand and you'll find there's not much you really can't join in with – just think about it first. You'll find that even split-second decisions can be made once you're really used to fitting diabetes into your social life.*

Chapter 9
REBELS WITH A CAUSE

Teenagers wouldn't be teenagers if they never tried to rebel. Whether it's playing loud music until all hours, making their own bizarre fashion statements or causing you sleepless nights worrying where they are, it comes with the territory! It's not easy trying to rationalize your adolescent's behaviour as the necessary rites of passage that will shape him into an adult when you are feeling stressed and anxious.

Whatever form your teenager's rebellion takes, diabetes is bound to come into the equation somewhere, either with the specific problems we've discussed earlier in this book (refusing to blood test/inject/eat and so on) or in more seemingly innocuous ways, such as disagreements over how to cope in certain situations. Siobhan – now 17 – told us:

My mother had always been very much against me having my ears pierced and I automatically assumed that the reason was because I had diabetes. She hadn't actually said this to me, but I'd heard somewhere that ear-piercing was not suitable for people with diabetes. So, when I was 15, to really give her something to scream about, I saved up my pocket money, went off and had them done. When I got home and made a big thing of defiantly showing them to her, I didn't get the reaction I'd expected. She just shrugged and said 'Well, you're old enough to make up your own mind now . . . I just didn't want you to have them done when you were younger and then regret it'. I called her a liar and said it was because of my diabetes that she hadn't wanted me to have my ears pierced. She laughed and said that was complete rubbish, she knew it was OK for people with diabetes to have it done. I felt really stupid!

We hope that we've helped some way towards solving certain problems relating directly to diabetes in other chapters. Below is a collection of 'problem page' queries posed by teenagers that, we hope, may sort out certain misunderstandings and family rows!

Fashion Statements

I've had my ears pierced, which was fine. Now, I'd like to have my nose and belly button done, too. My parents are shocked. Apart from the fact that they think it will look disgusting, they are convinced that having diabetes means I will get some dreadful infection. Is this true?
Jessie, 17.

All piercing should be carried out in a reputable establishment to ensure that equipment and so on is sterile. Never consider asking a friend to perform any piercing with a needle 'sterilized' under hot water or by naked flame.

Under the proper circumstances, the risk of infection after having your nose and belly button pierced is the same as that of having your ears pierced. Providing your diabetes is well-controlled and you follow the salon's hygiene instructions, you are no more likely to develop an infection than someone who does not have diabetes. However, if an infection should occur, follow the normal procedure of increasing insulin to cope with higher blood glucose levels and visit your GP as you may need antibiotics.

As for your parents' feelings about your piercing plans, why not wait a couple of months to make sure you really want to go through with it? This would also give them time to get used to the idea if you decide to go ahead.

I like wearing fashionable footwear, but I keep being told that I should wear very sensible shoes in case I get loss of feeling in my feet. My feet are fine and 'sensible shoes' are boring, so why should I take any notice? Saskia, 14.

The reason footcare is of great importance when you have diabetes is because you may begin to suffer from a complication called diabetic neuropathy (see Chapter 4), which is when the nerves in the feet may be affected, causing loss of feeling. If you wear shoes or boots that are tight (or too loose for that matter), causing blisters, bunions, corns and so on, then you may not feel any pain and, in time, this may cause problems if they become infected.

So-called 'sensible shoes' do not have to be unfashionable. Dr Martens, for instance, are designed to be comfortable and beneficial to the feet, and the same also applies to good makes of desert boots and different kinds of sports shoes, all of which seem to be enduringly fashionable.

The most important thing is that whatever you choose to wear on your feet must actually fit correctly. It's worth being measured properly and taking time when trying shoes to make sure they are the right size for your feet in both length and width so that no pinching or rubbing occurs. Even if you don't suffer from neuropathy, looking after your feet now could prevent trouble in the future.

I would like to have a tattoo on my upper arm. Is this safe when you have diabetes? Joe, 17.

The answer here is much the same as that given to the question above about body piercing. Remember, though, that whereas holes in the ears and so on will eventually close up if jewellery is not used, removing a tattoo is a painful and often unsuccessful business, which can cause scarring for life. If you must have a tattoo, make it a small one!

I've been arguing with my mum about having sunbed treatments. She seems to think that they are unsafe if you have diabetes. I can't see why. Please explain. Donna, 19.

Dermatologists do not regard sunbed treatments as completely safe for anyone, with or without diabetes. Sunbeds expose you to a very high level of UVA radiation, yet you are not supposed to wear sunscreens when you use one. A sunbed does not emit UVB rays (which cause skin to thicken slightly as a protective precaution), so your skin doesn't develop any natural defence and present research suggests overuse can cause skin cancer.

The reason your mother is worried is probably because heat can increase the absorption of insulin which in turn can lower blood glucose levels and cause hypos (this is why saunas, jacuzzis and so on carry warnings for people with diabetes). However, if you check glucose levels before and after going on a sunbed, then you will be able to see if the heat affects you in this way and lower your insulin accordingly for future treatments (and keep hypostoppers at hand just in case you need them). The same guidelines apply to hot weather in general. As far as looking tanned and healthy goes, there are so many excellent fake tanning products available, you might find it less time-consuming and expensive to use these lotions instead. When you want to tan in the sun, use a high-protection sunscreen to guard against premature ageing and the possibility of skin cancer later in life.

Holiday Help

I have been planning a gap year trip to India before university. There would be four of us, all the others male, but I'm getting into a lot of rows with my parents about this. They seem to think it's far too dodgy as far as medical facilities go and are convinced that I won't be able to find anything suitable to eat. I need to assure them that I'll survive. I'm not worried, so why should they be? Melanie, 18.

Your parents' attitude is understandable – after all, India is not around the corner and they won't be anywhere near you should problems arise. It's up to you to put their minds at rest. Show them that you are planning this trip in a responsible and mature way; that you are taking the travelling and the diabetes seriously.

Contact the BDA, which publishes a range of leaflets covering diabetes care in different countries (such as strength of insulin used there and so on) and lots of information on travelling in general. Speak to someone in the Dietary Department there about the kind of food you are likely to have and take their advice on planning your diet while you are there.

Always carry some form of glucose. If you haven't been too good about blood testing, start now and show your parents that you are serious about really looking after yourself and controlling your diabetes. Unfortunately, a gap year does not mean a gap from diabetes and the more drastic the change in environment, the more there is a need to find out how your blood glucose is affected. Use the checklist in Chapter 5 to work out what equipment to take and remember to carry insulin in a vacuum flask filled with melted ice, which prevents the insulin freezing, but keeps it cool.

Stomach upsets are very common to travellers in India, so you and your friends are quite likely to succumb to Delhi Belly. Contact the tourist board for a list of good hospitals in the areas you are visiting, and go to hospital sooner rather than later if you do have such problems. Also, make sure you take out adequate insurance that covers air ambulance return to the UK (advisable for everyone). Again, the BDA can help as it has its own insurance schemes.

As you can see, a trip to somewhere like India may not be as easy as you thought, but, with planning and serious consideration, it is likely to be successful and your parents are bound to be reassured if they can see you are planning responsibly.

My friends are all going to a three-day rock festival and I desperately want to join them. This is causing many arguments at home because my parents don't see how I can follow my diabetes routine. I think that I am perfectly capable of doing my injections and eating

(I'm on four injections a day) and I really can't see what the problem is. Robert, 16.

Rock festivals invariably mean sitting around for hours trapped in a sea of people – and that may mean not being able to get to the stalls selling food (which often have queues and expensive food when you do get there). The way round this would be to take masses of your own food and drink and keep it in a bag with you at all times. If you took advantage of those times when it *was* possible to get to the food stalls without a hassle (before you were sitting in the arena), then you could eat a hot meal. Veterans of rock festivals assure us all this is perfectly possible.

Testing blood glucose frequently would tell you how you were doing and you could adjust your insulin depending on the results. To be honest, the problems you might encounter concerning food at an English rock festival are not going to be as difficult as, say, trekking round India or the Australian outback! Don't pack your rucksack with clothes, use all the available space for non-perishable food and cartons of fruit juice, take enough money for extra meals and, as we've already advised, keep your bag with food, insulin and the rest with you at all times to avoid anything being stolen. There will, of course, be drugs available and we advise that you read Chapter 8, which explains why it's best to avoid anything offered.

We're going on a family trip to Australia, which involves a 24-hour flight with short stops. My father is insisting that I blood test every two hours, which seems ridiculous. I have refused to test as frequently as this and I'll admit that I'm not too hot on testing overall. How many times do you think I should test on the flight? My father also thinks I should order the in-flight diabetic meals, which I have also refused to do as I've heard they are unsuitable. I'm on four injections daily, with a pen. David, 15.

Any trip abroad has to be planned, and you are embarking on a very long-haul flight. Discuss flight times with your diabetes nurse and she will suggest a suitable injection regime. Your father is only showing his concern over testing and, as your diabetes nurse will tell you, it's important to blood test regularly during the flight as you may need to increase or decrease your insulin with all that sitting around and low-carbohydrate meals.

Show your father you are going to look after yourself by starting to test before meals and bedtime before you go. Start as you mean to go on and he will feel much happier about the whole thing! Don't bother to order the in-flight diabetic meal as these contain little or no carbohydrate – just order ordinary food and eat wisely. Also, take some extra carbohydrate with you, such as digestive biscuits.

A friend of mine who also has diabetes was recently searched at customs and accused of drug-taking because syringes were found in his bag. He showed the customs officer the insulin bottle, but this had little effect, even though he was found not to have any drugs on him. After a long hassle, they let him go, but the whole experience stressed him out. I'm going abroad soon for the first time since being diagnosed – how do I avoid this hassle? Charles, 17.

Carry a letter from your doctor stating that you have insulin-dependent diabetes (or an identity card from the BDA) and you shouldn't have a problem. Wear a bracelet or neck chain which states you have diabetes treated with insulin (SOS/Talisman or Medic-Alert jewellery are recognized worldwide symbols). However, having said all this, if you are found to be carrying illegal substances as well, you will have no case, so, no one should imagine they can use diabetes as a cover for carrying drugs!

My mum drives me crazy on holiday. I'm off having a great time with my friends and she searches me out at snack and mealtimes to remind me to eat. I am quite capable of sorting myself out, although I admit that sometimes I'm half an hour late or so and do start to feel hypo. I know she's concerned, but I wish she'd get off my back! Suzy, 12.

Of course it's annoying having someone interrupting your fun, but your mum has only got your best interests at heart. From what you say, she's got a point if you can't remember to eat at the right time and risk having a hypo. It's especially worrying when you're near water or swimming.

Wearing a watch that you can pre-set so an alarm beeps at snack times could be the answer. Then, you won't forget to eat, your mum will feel easier about the situation and leave you to be responsible for yourself, which, of course, you should be.

Emotional Times

I'm fed up with my parents nagging me about testing. They have told me over and over that unless I keep my blood sugar under good control, I will have all kinds of problems when I get older. I've had diabetes for three years and I've very rarely had good figures. As I see it now, life won't be worth living in a few years anyway, so what's the point of struggling with blood tests? It seems like a waste of time to me. Gary, 16.

What you're actually saying is that you simply want to roll over and accept something you regard as inevitable. In Chapter 4, we talked about diabetic complications and how the risks can be *lessened* by good control. So, nothing is inevitable, but your input is vital in this particular situation. Diabetes is your condition and while you say that you are fed up with your parents nagging, consider their feelings. Because the situation is in your hands, they have to stand by and watch the son they love do his best to self-destruct.

Instead of being so negative, try to see that you have everything to stay fit and healthy for. It's certainly not too late to get to grips with your diabetes now. Once you achieve better control, you are bound to feel better physically and this should hopefully give you the spur to carry on and shake off this negative attitude.

I get periods of feeling very angry with life. I can't say that my diabetes stops me doing anything, but sometimes the thought of having it overwhelms me. When I get these feelings, I get into arguments at home and trouble at school. I don't want to be like this, but I don't

seem to be able to get out of these moods once they come over me.
Steve, 15.

There is nothing unusual about being angry because you have diabetes. However, as you have said yourself, the way you are generating that anger is the real problem.

Anger is a very physical emotion and can be turned into something good. Using up that aggressive energy in sport, for instance, can have very positive results. If you feel like hitting someone, why not install a punchbag in your room and take any aggression out on that? Anger expressed in a creative way – such as writing, drawing or painting – can be powerful and rewarding. There are countless musicians who have expressed their darker emotions in song. For example, Beethoven's music often expressed his despair at being deaf.

Try to talk openly to others, too. Diabetes is not a taboo subject and it's nothing to be ashamed of. Sharing your feelings and confiding in those you are close to can only have positive results.

I'm very upset about something my mother did which I regard as a complete betrayal of trust. I have a boyfriend called Tim, and we've been seeing each other for a month. I didn't tell Tim I had diabetes as I was afraid it would put him off me. My mother knew this and, one night when he came to pick me up, she told him while I was getting ready. He took it really well, but seemed annoyed that the information had come from my mother. I did not want Tim to know until I felt ready to tell him myself and I feel very angry that she has let me down. Sally, 16.

We can see why Tim was irritated that he had to hear the news from your mother, but we can also understand why she felt compelled to tell him (although perhaps she could have warned you that she was going to, thus giving you the chance to tell him yourself). Not telling someone who is spending time with you that you have diabetes and may require help if a potentially dangerous situation arises is, frankly, unfair on them. Knowing that you have diabetes obviously didn't put Tim off you, as you still refer to him as your boyfriend. If it had done, surely he wouldn't have been worth carrying on with anyway? Make the peace with your mum – she was only acting in your best interests.

Whenever I've been invited to a party there's a row. My parents say that I can't go because I won't be able to eat the food, then I'll have a hypo and make myself ill. When this happens I lock myself in my room and refuse to do my insulin injections so I can make myself ill anyway. It's not fair, none of my friends have this problem and I'm missing out on all the fun. Alice, 13.

Diabetes can be used as an emotional weapon – and not just by the person who actually has it. Is there an underlying reason for your parents being so against you going to these parties? Are they concerned about the people you are mixing with, lack of parental control or do they imagine there will be drinking and/or drug-taking?

By refusing to take your insulin, you are using the same weapon as your parents, namely your diabetes.

While we can see your point, two wrongs don't make a right. If you really feel that they are being unreasonable and that the party in question is above board and fulfils the requirements that any concerned parent of a young teenager could wish for, try discussing the situation calmly and allay their fears so that they give you the chance to prove that you will be fine. Perhaps you could suggest they phone the parents of the friend who is holding the party to put their minds at rest. As for the food, there is bound to be carbohydrate available (pizza, crisps, French bread and so on are staple party foods for teenagers), but if you really want to stop them worrying about your eating, have a meal before you go. Show them that you carry glucose tablets at all times, take a bottle of diet cola and agree to phone them sometime during the evening.

I think I'm old enough to go to the diabetes clinic alone, but my mother insists on coming along. I think it's embarrassing, especially as she often answers the questions that the diabetes nurse asks me, as if I'm not there. At what age do you think it's right to go for check-ups without parents? Jill, 15.

Until you are 16, you are your parents' responsibility with regard to medical matters. However, doctors treat patients as individuals and do not automatically see all young people with their parents.

If you find the situation embarrassing, try to discuss how you feel with your mum. Suggest that you see a doctor or nurse on your own while she waits outside and then invite her into the room when you have finished talking so she can have her say. She will get used to the idea eventually, and will surely be reassured when she realizes that you want to take responsibility for your diabetes. Perhaps your mother has a problem with letting go (see Chapter 10 for more on how other parents cope).

I've heard the term 'brittle diabetes'. Can you tell me what this means as my blood sugars are up and down and I wonder whether it applies to me. Jonathan, 18.

Brittle diabetes is a term that is often misleadingly used to describe diabetes which is difficult to control. Of course, diabetes is difficult to control at times and sugar levels do rise and fall, but the difference between this and brittle diabetes is that people with the latter are frequently admitted to hospital with either very high or low blood glucose. Even though their diabetes is then stabilized and they go home, it's not long before they are back in hospital again.

Essentially, this is an emotional problem rather than an actual physical one and tends to be more common in teenage girls, who may need counselling. Fortunately, with maturity and emotional stability, hospital admissions diminish and brittle diabetes usually goes away.

Eating Habits

I'm on two injections a day and I'm getting fed up with having to remember between-meal snacks, let alone eat them. I often miss them out, which leads to feeling hypo well before the main meal is due. I've heard that multiple injections of short-acting insulin would free me from all this and that I could even miss meals out if I felt like it.

However, I've also heard that there's more chance of gaining weight on four injections a day. Please could you fill me in on the correct information? Sarah, 16.

You are quite right in thinking that a four-times-a-day regime could add flexibility to your life and may eliminate the need for some snacks. However, we would stress that you discuss this in detail with your diabetes nurse and dietitian so that they understand your aims and can take your reduced food intake into account when working out your new regime.

This said, no insulin regime takes away the need for regular meals. While you may be able to delay the timing of a meal should you need to, it should only be the exception rather than the rule that you actually miss a meal and injection completely (perhaps an all-night party has meant you have slept for much of the following day, making it impossible to have too many meals on top of each other), otherwise your diabetes will become uncontrollable.

There's no reason for you to gain weight if you do multiple injections, providing you are sensible with your food intake and are not always increasing your insulin to allow you to eat more fattening foods. Talk the whole thing through with your diabetes care team so that any problems can be sorted out immediately, should they arise.

I'm on four injections a day and I eat quite sensibly. Sometimes, though, I'm out with my friends and they want to eat chocolate between meals and, to be honest, so do I. Should I give myself an extra shot of insulin to cover this? Beverly, 18.

Providing the rest of your diet is sensible, there is no reason for you not to include some chocolate as a treat sometimes. Try to ration the amount you eat a little bit so as not to upset your blood glucose too much. But, by all means, join in with your friends. However, if this is to be a daily habit, consider having an alternative snack, such as cereal bars or crisps on some days – don't give extra insulin to cover chocolate between meals as the rise in your blood glucose will not coincide with your insulin and you may end up feeling hypo later on.

> *I go out drinking quite a lot, much to my parents displeasure. There is always a dispute about my eating beforehand, which, frankly, I don't want to do. Everyone else has a meal in the pub or wine bar, usually after a few drinks. Do I have to eat before I start drinking or is it acceptable to eat during or after the session?* Paul, 18.

Drinking on an empty stomach is asking for trouble as alcohol can have a very unpredictable effect on blood glucose, causing you to have a hypo before you know it (and leaving your friends with the task of having to bring you round!) Having an extra snack beforehand (or as you reach the pub) is the best way to avoid this. A sandwich or roll should be plenty. You can then join in with the meal as usual later on. It's also a good idea to have the odd soft drink or fruit juice to spread the alcohol out (while still being seen to be drinking!)

Your parents realize they will not stop you drinking, but are trying to prevent you from getting into a potentially dangerous situation. By causing a scene over eating beforehand, you are making them feel you are not yet responsible enough to go out drinking. Having a hypo while out will simply give them the chance to say, 'We told you so!' and make them even more worried!

> *Ever since I was diagnosed as having diabetes six years ago, my mother has religiously measured my portions of food. I even have my own cereal bowl with a line drawn showing where the Shreddies should stop! This seems ridiculous to me and it's very annoying because she stops me having second helpings or anything extra. I have a friend with diabetes who eats the amount he wants and no one in his family makes a fuss. My mother is unimpressed by this and it's driving me crazy as I'm starving hungry most of the time as well as feeling pretty hard done by. What do you think I should do?*
> Tom, 13.

Your mum is trying very hard to keep your diabetes under control by watching your diet, but she seems to have got her messages a little confused. As you grow, you are bound to need more food and the fact that you are starving hungry proves this.

The best way to approach your mum is to tell her just how hungry you are and suggest that you both go and see the dietitian, who can suggest more suitable quantities of food. This will give you the opportunity to ask about things like second helpings and your mum can mention things that are worrying her. The chances are, she will be relieved to find that she doesn't have to be so strict! But, going on to her about what your friend does is not a good way to tackle things because he is not necessarily right either. There's always a good compromise between eating too much and too little.

Chapter 10

LETTING GO

If your child has had diabetes for some time, the chances are that once the teenage years arrive you will more or less have consigned injections, blood tests, decisions about insulin, food and so on to him. Yet, while your teenager is still living under your roof, at least you have a window on what's going on and, to a large extent, can keep a subtle eye on things. How will you feel, though, when your child leaves the nest? As many elderly parents of middle-aged men or women will testify, their offspring are – to them – still their 'babies' and however ably your son or daughter appears to be coping with diabetes control, you may be dreading the day they depart for pastures new, away from your ever-watchful eye. One mother says:

I dreaded the day Robert was due to go off to a job in London where he would be sharing a flat. It was irrational really, he'd coped so well for a long time, but I'd always been in the background. For the first few months I carried a mobile phone around wherever I went. Of course, he only called me once a week on a Sunday. He said he was fine . . . But I imagined he was hiding all sorts of things from me. Gradually, though, I relaxed and left the mobile phone at home. He's been away for three years now and is getting married soon to a lovely girl. I'll still worry though.

Anne's daughter, Victoria, is at university:

When Victoria lived at home, we tended to check whether she'd had her injections, snacks, etc. if she was staying with friends. Now, it's all under her control. We're concerned that she drinks too much, but she tells us she manages to avoid hypos by eating before going to bed. We try very hard to stop worrying about what she is getting up to and we make it clear that we're here if she needs us and will pay for her fare home. She actually did come home last week because she was run-down with a tooth abscess.

Laura's mother, Susan, says:

She'll be leaving soon to go to university. I'll worry the same amount as I did when her older sister went three years ago. But I know she'll be fine.

The key to letting go of your child is to make it clear right from the start (as soon as they are able to understand, in the case of young children) that it is *his* diabetes, not *yours*. He is the person who must ultimately become responsible for his treatment and his own actions. Once he takes this on board, he is well on the way to becoming independent of you.

Most children who were diagnosed as having diabetes prior to being a teenager tend to reach a point where they are only too pleased to take matters into their own hands so that they can join in with their friends and lead a normal life without parental interference. Those who develop diabetes in the teens should be encouraged to take responsibility right from the beginning and start as they mean to go on.

However much you still see them as vulnerable children, it won't be that long before they will want to leave the nest – not that many 20-somethings willingly live at home! It's true, however, that some parents can – with the best will in the world – be so over-protective that the child continues to have his diabetes controlled by a parent well into adolescence. As Mick (now 18) told us:

I didn't realize how little responsibility I actually had . . . the years had just passed without me noticing that at the age of 15 I was still carrying on as if I was a young kid. I automatically cut short evenings out to go home and have my injection and meal. I just did it . . . but I was getting pretty damn fed up with it.

I mentioned this to my diabetes nurse; she was quite shocked. She asked me why I didn't take my insulin out with me and just get on with it. I replied that my mother had always expected me home and it was a habit. The nurse had a long chat with Mum, who was genuinely upset that she seemed to have been curtailing my lifestyle, even though it was more by habit than design.

I could tell she was fearful the first time I wasn't coming home for dinner, but she got used to it in the end. I can kind of understand why she was so overprotective . . . but my advice is the earlier you do everything yourself, the better or you become cocooned.

As you will see later in this chapter, BDA holidays are a fantastic way of giving your teenager a taste of early independence before he launches out into the world of trips without the watchful eyes of adults trained in the treatment of diabetes. School trips taken from an early age (sometimes in the last years of primary school) give the child a chance to take over his diabetes management, and he is bound to be keen to do everything right so that he's not a millstone around anyone's neck. In fact, he will probably be extra-careful to make sure he looks after his diabetes perfectly.

Provide the teacher in charge with a duplicate set of equipment (injection device, insulin, blood test strips, glucose and so on) and a checklist of instructions in the event of emergency. Have a chat about your child's requirements and, hopefully, everything will go smoothly. In this case, your child should be capable of drawing up insulin or assembling and using his pen, interpreting blood test results and acting accordingly. Linda told us:

Anna is about to go off on a week's trip to Scotland with the school. She's 11. I'll admit that I'm very apprehensive in some ways, but I'm also excited for her – she's got it all worked out and she's determined to have a great time. She doesn't want to be ill while she's there, so I feel confident that she'll do everything right.

If your child hasn't tasted real freedom by the time he reaches secondary school age, this will almost certainly be the time he wants to go out and about with friends, unencumbered by adults. Despite the fact that we as parents fear the dangers of the outside world in general, we owe it to our children to give them independence when they are ready. There is no reason for a youngster not to go out with friends before he is a fully-fledged teenager *if* he can be trusted to be responsible and mature. The age at which such maturity develops varies with each individual and therefore it's impossible to give a definite age when a child will be ready to take unaccompanied train journeys, shopping expeditions and so on, but whether a child has diabetes or not, you would probably not be happy to have him on the loose if he were young for his years. On the other hand, a child who can be trusted to act in a responsible way will benefit from being given responsibility for himself from an earlier age.

One condition most parents give is that the youngster phones them at a designated time and, most importantly, if he is going to be arriving home later than he originally said that another phonecall is made to explain that he missed the bus/the film ended later than he thought/the shopping trip lasted longer than planned. Don't give them any excuse not to call – give them a phonecard or BT chargecard (preferably programmed to only connect with your home number) rather than loose change for public phones as this has a mysterious way of being spent on other things.

Suzy was just 11 when she asked the vet if she could help out with the animals on a Sunday. I arranged to pick her up at lunchtime and sent her along with a mid-morning snack. Later that morning, she phoned and asked if she could stay to watch some operations. It was a fantastic chance for her, but she didn't have any food for lunch. I offered to take something to her, but that went down like a lead balloon. 'I'll sort it out myself', she said. I felt pretty apprehensive, wondering whether she'd bother to eat at all. Would she faint from a hypo rather than the gore of the operations? But, when I picked her up later that afternoon, she had borrowed some money from the vet's nurse, gone to the shop and bought a sandwich and orange juice to get her through. 'I can look after myself, Mum', she told me. Now, so long as she always carries ID and glucose tablets when she's out, I believe her.

Of course, we as parents are bound to worry far more than the teenager themselves – they are used to living with diabetes and we are only observers from the outside. When John (in his late teens) went on his first holiday abroad with 'the lads', his mum, Barbara, went through hell:

I found it impossible to think it all through . . . the journeys, the meals, all those requirements . . . I was extremely apprehensive before he went (to say the least!) and I imagined all sorts of terrible things happening to him. Yet, I knew he had to go off without us sometime and I gradually relaxed after he'd been gone for a few days and the police hadn't knocked at the door . . . He did, of course, survive without us and is very keen to go off again.

One anxious mum reports:

Gemma is about to embark on a gap year back-pack around India. I really don't know how I'm going to survive the worrying, but I know she's got to do it. Apart from the fact that she can't wait to go, she needs this opportunity to prove that she can branch out on her own and, in my heart of hearts, I know she'll cope.

Sometimes leaving home is just what the teenager needs to push him into taking real responsibility for his diabetes:

Our son's drinking affected our life most. It was a constant worry while he lived at home. He also neglected his diabetes regime and we've always felt we have to support him more than our other children. However, he certainly seems to be acting more sensibly on both the drinking and the diabetes now he has moved into his own home. We still worry an awful lot about him eating sensibly and we find it hard to settle if he does not contact us regularly.

Sarah, aged 17, is now at boarding school. Her mother, Jenny, says:

I feel that boarding for the sixth form is a good halfway house to leaving home for university.

Another mum voices what is a general consensus of opinion:

You don't relish the thought of them leaving home for any length of time. We've been through umpteen school trips, a gap year trek round Europe and now a flat-share with three other lads who appear to be totally disorganized, but, still, what can you do? You just have to get a grip on yourself and let go.

Sometimes parents underestimate the effect that diabetes has on a child's maturity. Many youngsters who on the surface seem rather gauche or childish are actually far more mature deep down than they would have you think.

Sally can be quite crazy and seemingly feckless in many ways, yet, beneath it all, there's a strong character who is in charge of herself and her diabetes. It's certainly been character-building for her. I know that if there's a crisis, she's the strong one.

Sezen, 16, recognizes this strength of character in herself:

The positive aspect of my diabetes was learning to take care of myself. Being my own doctor, feeling more independent . . . Before, I used to count on my parents to do things for me . . . I was a sort of 'mummy's girl'. But the diabetes helped me build up a mature character pretty fast!

So, surely the conclusion has to be, when your teenager wants to spread his wings, let him do so willingly. Anxiety is only natural, but try keeping it on the inside and trust him. When he leaves home, perhaps you could present him with a good luck card with the following messages.

- Feel free to enjoy your new life without me sticking my oar in!
- You may not be able to imagine it, but I was a teenager once and sometimes my advice and experience just might be worth some attention!
- Find yourself a doctor and new diabetes team to take over your care and keep your appointments!
- Please tell me if you have any problems. I don't expect you to come running home every two minutes, but I want to help, whatever the problem.
- Keep in contact – there's nothing worse than not hearing regularly from someone you love.

BDA Holidays

One overriding factor that was mentioned over and over again in our survey of teenagers was the positive effects of BDA activities. These vary from get-together weekends to outward bound holidays, watersports and skiing trips (there are various holidays for different age groups). Children can enjoy these breaks from the age of five and continue into their late teens if they so wish.

The real bonus of these trips (especially for younger children) is that they are run by doctors and nurses who specialize in diabetes, and youngsters learn from each other. Many parents report younger children going to camp unwilling to do their own injections and coming home experts in the technique. For teenagers, the chance to take part in all sorts of hair-raising activities that they might never otherwise have tried can be irresistible. Judy, now 16, says:

I've been going year after year. I don't think I'd ever have had the chance – or dared – to do half the things I've done on those trips. It's good to share experiences with others in the same position as yourself. It gives you belief in your own abilities for later on.

Sarah says:

I've taken part in two adventure weekends in Wales, doing abseiling, canoeing and rock-climbing, which was excellent fun. Knowing that so many others had diabetes gave me the confidence to do everything and get to know lots of people I wouldn't otherwise have met.

Christopher had his first taste of skiing in France with the BDA when he was 13:

It was an excellent introduction to the sport and when I went with the school the following year, not only could I cope easily with my diabetes, I could also ski better than most of the others!

If your child is interested in a BDA holiday – and be warned, they get booked up pretty quickly! – contact the Youth Department at the BDA (see the Useful Addresses section at the back of this book).

Chapter 11

A CURE – FACT
OR FICTION?

However settled your teenager may be in her diabetes regime, it is only natural that you are on the look-out for any new developments in the search for an actual cure. Every so often, the media trumpets new breakthroughs that raise your hopes, only to end in disappointment when you discover that the information given has been hyped up and blown out of all proportion.

Unfortunately, the simple answer is that there is no cure at present. However, doctors and scientists continue to study diabetes and work towards that ultimate achievement. Vast sums of money are poured into these efforts and one day it will happen.

Hopefully, this will be in your child's lifetime, but, until such a time, we should be content and grateful for advances in technology that make living with diabetes easier than ever before. Gadgets become smaller, faster, simpler and less intrusive than ever. Needles are shorter and finer, injection devices are user-friendly and disposable, glucose meters are miniature hi-tech miracles. When you think that bulky glass syringes and urine testing skills were the norm 20 or so years ago, you can see just how far we've come!

Painless Monitoring?

We talked about the possibility of infra-red blood glucose readings replacing finger-prickers in Chapter 3, and this does, indeed, look like becoming a reality. Most of the research is being carried out in America and one company has been the first to submit its version of a sensor to the US Food and Drug Administration (FDA). It now awaits approval being granted. There are a number of other companies looking into this development and it is generally agreed that sensors will become available in the future.

In the meanwhile, there are problems. The infra-red beam has to pass through skin, bone, muscle and the walls of the blood vessels, which may affect the reading. Temperature and sweating present problems, too. Also, each individual's skin is a different thickness, so a beam that may detect the blood glucose level in a child may not work on an adult. The device also has to be small enough to be carried in a pocket or worn as a wristwatch. One further important consideration is that it must be cost-effective. It is pointless producing a meter that enables blood glucose monitoring to be painless when it is financially out of reach of most people with diabetes. However, technology is becoming so advanced that these problems are likely to be overcome in the not-too-distant future.

Nasal Insulin

Ever since the discovery of insulin, there has been much interest in trying to find a way to administer it other than by injection. As insulin is a protein, it cannot be taken by mouth as it is digested before it has any effect. There has, however, been a great deal of interest in nasal insulin.

Researchers were faced with the problem that the insulin molecule is too large to cross through the nasal membrane and be absorbed into the bloodstream. Scientists then added 'enhancers', which supposedly helped absorption. Unfortunately, these were not successful and the insulin still could not pass through the nasal membrane into the bloodstream.

The search went on for an an effective enhancer and, now, at Temple University in Philadelphia, they think they have the answer – liquorice! Forget liquorice sweets, this enhancer is actually *essence* of liquorice. Trials have been carried out and the results lead scientists to believe that this works, so larger trials are now being undertaken.

Those who support the research say nasal insulin could be given *before* meals, allowing it to be absorbed quicker to coincide with the carbohydrate intake. However, there are those who say nasal insulin can never replace insulin injections and Temple University still has a long way to go before it can even gain approval from the FDA to allow the further trials that would be necessary before a nasal spray could go on the market.

Pumps

We mentioned a device in Chapter 3 that provides a continuous flow of insulin, known as a continuous subcutaneous insulin infusion pump. At one time, there was much enthusiasm for these – at least from doctors. These pumps have never replaced insulin injections for many reasons, including that patients did not like them as much as was anticipated and there were all sorts of problems with leakages and infection. They are sometimes used when tight control is vital (as in pregnancy), but, apart from special circumstances, they have not been found to be a viable alternative to injections.

Over the last 20 years or so, research into implantable insulin pumps has progressed slowly. Now there are a couple of pumps that look promising. These are disk-shaped, 7 to 9 cm in diameter and 1.9 to 2.5 cm thick (2¾ to 3½ in by ¾ to 1 in) and must be inserted into the left-hand side of the abdomen under anaesthetic. A tube is attached, through which insulin is delivered by timed pulses. At the time of writing, trials of these pumps are in progress and they are being compared to multiple insulin injection regimes. However, the main problem is that the tubing becomes blocked with small amounts of tissue. This can be removed, but involves a minor surgical procedure.

These types of pumps are in the research stage at the moment, but, if you think such an implant sounds too far-fetched, think again – no doubt people greeted the first news of pacemakers with disbelief, too!

Transplants

Diabetes is caused by the failure of the beta cells in the pancreas, so, surely, the answer is to simply transplant the pancreas. After all, kidney transplants, for example, are commonplace now. Unfortunately, pancreas transplants are not as successful as those of the kidney.

The first pancreas transplant was carried out in 1966. The result was not good because the digestive enzymes produced by the pancreas digested the surrounding tissues in the unknown environment. In the late 1970s, scientists discovered a way of killing off the digestive enzymes but not the beta cells, so, when the pancreas was transplanted, only the beta cells would function.

Although a successful pancreas transplant does mean that the person with diabetes then has normal blood glucose and does not need insulin, quite often the body eventually rejects the new pancreas, so the procedure cannot be said to be an answer to our prayers.

One significant problem with a transplant is the need for immunosuppressive medication. The body has its own defence mechanisms against anything 'foreign', which is how it fights infection. So, when any donor organ (a pancreas in this case) is transplanted, the body's defence mechanism goes into action and attacks the new pancreas, aiming to destroy it. To combat this, the person who has a transplanted organ must take medication to prevent rejection. However, these drugs have side-effects. They weaken the ability of the immune system to fight infection and can make the patient more susceptible to certain cancers. Because of the side-effects of the medication, pancreas transplants are carried out only in those who also need a kidney transplant. This makes sense as immunosuppressive medication has to be taken anyway to prevent the kidney from being rejected. However such double transplants are not always the answer as kidney and pancreas transplants have a higher rate of failure than kidney-only transplants.

The real alternative to pancreas transplants must surely be islet cell transplants. As it is the islet cells that are needed to produce insulin, surely only these need to be transplanted? Initially, scientists were faced with the problem of how to separate the cells from the pancreas. At first, the only way to do this was to put a dissected pancreas under a microscope and remove the islets. Then, in the 1960s, a way was found to separate the islets by using an enzyme to digest the surrounding tissue. But, although islet transplantation does not require major surgery (they can be injected through a vein or placed under the skin), there is still the problem of rejection and so immunosuppressants have to be taken.

Scientists are working on ways of getting round this. One way is to place the cells in a type of tubing that is compatible with the body. The tubing protects the islets from being destroyed, but allows them to react to glucose. Research is continuing into the material from which such tubes are made. It is important that the tube does not move within the body or it will be seen as a foreign object and be surrounded by a coat of fibrous tissue, preventing it from working. There is also the problem of how many islets are needed and how long they can survive for.

Another way of trying to prevent the islets from being destroyed is to encapsulate them in tiny beads or a membrane, then place them in a body cavity or inject them into a vein so they will go directly to the liver. The idea is that insulin could then pass out of the membrane or bead, yet antibodies would not be able to go in. With this method, there are the same problems of rejection, how many islets need to be transplanted and how long they will survive.

Then there is the added problem of donors. It can take up to three pancreases to provide enough islets for one person requiring a transplant. However, if encapsulating islet cells is successful, animal islets (probably pig) would have to be used as demand would outweigh supply. At present, few people who have had islet transplants have actually been able to come off insulin. Also, although pancreas transplants have come a long way since the 1960s, more research is needed into transplantation, and this continues.

Genetics

At the time of writing, a major research project into finding who is likely to develop insulin-dependent diabetes is underway. There is a genetic susceptibility to developing diabetes, but not everyone who is susceptible will actually go on to have diabetes. Therefore, there must be environmental factors that trigger off diabetes. If this is the case, then perhaps by changing the environment or using some kind of drug intervention before or at the early stage of beta cell damage, diabetes could be prevented.

It appears that environmental factors play a part in the development of the condition because the incidence rate of insulin-dependent diabetes in several countries is seasonal. Also, in only 36 per cent of cases do identical twins both develop diabetes, so, although they are genetically identical, for some reason an environmental factor will act as a trigger in one and not the other. Viral infections, diet, infection and lifestyle are being looked at, but at the moment no common factors have been found.

A big problem is that 90 per cent of people with insulin-dependent diabetes have no immediate family history of it and, therefore, there is no way scientists can tell who will develop diabetes using hereditary factors (unless, of course, the entire population were to be screened). However, there have been some advances in genetics as researchers have been able to analyse 23 pairs of chromosomes in about 600 people with a family history of diabetes.

We get our chromosomes from our parents. These, in turn, are made up of long chains of deoxyribonucleic acid – more commonly known as DNA – and we each have 100,000 pairs of genes. We already know of two genes – IDDM1 and IDDM2 – that contribute to an individual developing diabetes, but, as yet, the environmental trigger factor remains elusive. Two more genes – IDDM4 and IDDM5 – have also been found, but, as yet, researchers are not clear as to exactly what part they play in the development of diabetes. IDDM1 is the most important of these genes, but even that does not cause diabetes in every case, so more research needs to be done before a cure can be found.

So Where Does This Leave Us?

Comparing what you have just read to the hyped up media stories of cures may make you feel despondent, and the pace of research seems achingly slow when you are impatient for a cure for your child. Yet, it's more than likely that, with all that's going on, there *will* be a major breakthrough in the not-too-distant future. In the meantime, consider just how far the treatment for diabetes has progressed since insulin was discovered in the 1920s and remember that diabetes – even though it is a complicated balancing act – is, at the end of the day, a treatable condition. One mother recalls her thoughts on this:

> *When Sophie was a difficult teenager, I used to have this recurring dream that a cure had been found – a simple operation or something and that would be that. But, I'd wake up and the nightmare went on. Sophie was so irresponsible I honestly doubted that she'd make it through her teens. Now I can tell you that she's 30 with a couple of lovely children, a model mother and wife who also has a career. We've come out the other end and it's all a blur. How did she get through her teens? How did we get through her teens? Don't ask me – we just did it!*

BIBLIOGRAPHY

British Diabetic Association information and literature

Brook Advisory Centre information on teenage pregnancy and contraception

Cohen, Julian, and Kay, James, *Taking Drugs Seriously*, London, Thorsons, 1994

Department of Health, *Drug and Solvent Misuse*, London, Department of Health, 1993

Department of Health, *Solvents – A Parent's Guide*, London, Department of Health, 1993

Healey, Tim, and Fodoor, Mary, *History of the Diabetic Diet*, Toronto, University of Toronto Press, 1992

Health Education Authority, *Smoking – The Facts*, London, Health Education Authority, 1991

USEFUL ADDRESSES

British Diabetic Association (BDA)
10 Queen Anne Street
London W1M 0BD
Tel: *0171–323 1531*

• National organization providing links between people who have diabetes and their families and publishing the latest information on care and treatment. Also, invaluable advice on insurance, travelling, diet and local support groups.

BAPS Publications Unit
DSS Distribution Centre
Heywood Stores
Manchester Road
Heywood
Lancashire OL10 2P2

• Department of Health literature on drugs and solvents available from them.

The Advisory Council on Alcohol and Drug Education
(TACADE)
1 Hulme Place
The Crescent
Salford
Greater Manchester M5 4QA
Tel: *0161–745 8925*

• Literature and advice available from them.

Brook Advisory Centre
Central Office
233 Tottenham Court Road
London W1P 9AE
Tel: *0171–323 1522*

• They provide counselling, medical advice and literature on sexual matters.

Health Education Authority
Hamilton House
Mabledon Place
London WC1H 9TX
Tel: *0171–383 3833*

• It provides literature and advice on all aspects of smoking, drinking and drugs.

Bayer Diagnostics UK
Ames Division
Evans House
Hamilton Close
Basingstoke
Hampshire RG21 2YE
Tel: *01256 29181*

• Makers of blood glucose testing equipment.

Boehringer Mannheim UK
Bell Lane
Lewes
East Sussex BN7 1LG
Tel: *01273 480444*

• Manufacturers of blood testing equipment, they will supply starter packs and literature.

MediSense Britain Limited
17 The Courtyard
Gorsey Lane
Coles Hill
Birmingham B46 1JA
Tel: *01675 467044*

• They produce Exactech and MediSense blood testing equipment, including a pen sensor that particularly appeals to teenagers.

Owen Mumford Limited
Brook Hill
Woodstock
Oxford OX7 1TU
Tel: *01993 812021*

• Contact them for a brochure that includes blood glucose testing equipment, accessories and all kinds of carrying equipment.

Becton Dickinson
Between Towns Road
Cowley
Oxford OX4 3LY
Tel: *01865 777722*

• Manufacturers and suppliers of needles and syringes.

Eli Lilly and Company Limited
Kingsclere Road
Basingstoke
Hampshire RG21 6XA
Tel: *01256 315000*

• Insulin manufacturers who produce 'fun' pens for youngsters.

Novo Nordisk Pharmaceuticals Limited
Novo Nordisk House
Broadfield Park
Brighton Road
Pease Pottage
Crawley
West Sussex RH11 9RT
Tel: *01293 613555*

• Insulin manufacturers who operate a special youth scheme that teenagers can join. They also manufacture insulin pens and needles.

Medic-Alert Foundation
12 Bridge Wharf
156 Caledonian Road
London N1 9RD
Tel: *0171–833 3034*

• Makers of identification jewellery that carries engraved condition and central phone number information for relevant individual details.

SOS/Talisman
Golden Key Company Limited
1 Hare Street
Sheerness
Kent ME12 1AH

• Makers of identification jewellery with a special range of medallions depicting favourite sports.

INDEX

Of further interest...

Recipes for Health: Diabetes

Low fat, low sugar, carbohydrate-counted recipes
for the management of diabetes

Azmina Govindji and Jill Myers

This imaginative cookbook is also a comprehensive guide to living with diabetes, containing practical information as well as a delicious range of over 100 recipes carefully devised for a diabetic diet. It includes easy, everyday meals, meals for two, recipes to entertain with, ideas for cooking for children, vegetarian meals, tempting desserts and much more.

Each recipe is coded for calories and carbohydrate content. The recipes are ideal for anyone wanting a healthy low fat, high fibre, low sugar diet.